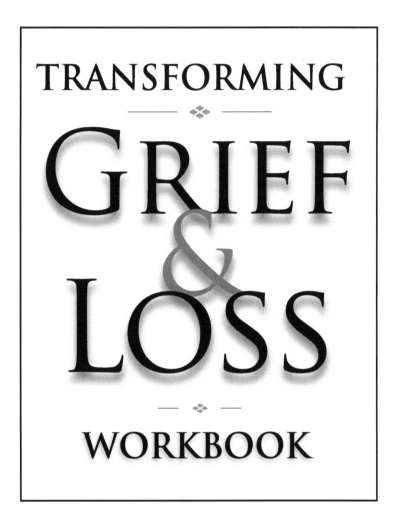

TRANSFORMING

GRIEF & LOSS

WORKBOOK

LIGIA M. HOUBEN, MA, FT, CGC, CPC, CHT

Creator of The 11 Principles of Transformation®

From the bottom of my heart I give thanks to Linda Jackson for giving me the opportunity to write this book. I am grateful for my supportive husband and for all who helped me in one way or another to make this book a reality. My deepest gratitude goes to my amazing clients and the participants of my seminars and workshops. They inspire me to continue with my mission of helping others transform their loss and transform their lives.

With all my love, this book is dedicated to the memory of my beloved father,
Julio C. Martinez A.

He was the inspiration for creating The 11 Principles of Transformation®
My father lives in my heart.

Copyright © 2017 by Ligia M. Houben

Published by:
PESI Publishing & Media
PESI, Inc
3839 White Ave
Eau Claire, WI 54703

Cover: Amy Rubenzer
Editing: Bookmasters
Layout: Bookmasters & Amy Rubenzer

ISBN: 9781683730026

Proudly printed in the United States of America

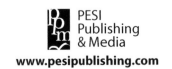

www.pesipublishing.com

ABOUT THE AUTHOR

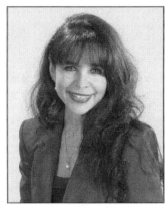

Ligia M. Houben, MA, FT, FAAGC, CPC, CHt, is the founder of My Meaningful Life, LLC and of The Center for Transforming Lives in Miami, where she consults with individuals and families through coaching groups, workshops, meditation and yoga classes. Ligia is a whole-hearted speaker in the field of grief, loss, life transitions and personal growth.

She is an international speaker and has appeared on numerous radio and television programs, including CNN Español, NPR, NBC, and Univisión. A pioneer in working with Hispanics and grief, she authored the book *Counseling Hispanics through Loss, Grief, and Bereavement: A Guide for Mental Health Professionals*, which has been widely embraced as a helping manual in clinical settings, hospitals, and individuals.

Ligia is former board member of The Association for Death, Education, and Counseling (ADEC), is a Fellow in Thanatology and a Fellow in the American Academy of Grief Counseling. She is a Certified Grief Counselor, Thanatologist, Counselor, and Professional Coach (CPC). Through PESI, she presents her signature seminar *Transforming Grief & Loss: Strategies to Help your Clients through Major Life Transitions*, based on Houben's The 11 Principles of Transformation®, the system she created to transform losses into personal growth and introduced in her self-help book *Transform Your Loss: Your Guide to Strength and Hope*.

She holds a BA in psychology and religious studies from the University of Miami, MA in religious studies and graduate certificates in multidisciplinary gerontology from Florida International University, and in loss and healing from St. Thomas University.

TABLE OF CONTENTS

INTRODUCTION

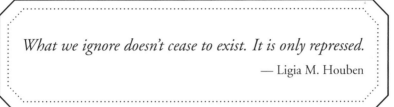

> *What we ignore doesn't cease to exist. It is only repressed.*
> — Ligia M. Houben

We all experience losses in our lives. Your clients experience losses. You also experience losses. And although it is common and natural, we are not educated or trained to deal with losses. We live in a death-denial society that at times forces us to suppress our feelings regarding major life transitions and continue living as if nothing happened. It is not possible, because what matters most is not to ignore what has happened to us, but to find ways to transform what has happened to us. Therefore, you will find the tendency of this workbook to be hopeful, positive, and empowering, as it offers valuable tools and life skills that will help your clients transform their loss and transform their lives.

Let's keep in mind that happiness is a state we all desire. As Judith Belmont stated, *"Regardless of mental health discipline or training background, it is safe to say that we all share a common goal with our clients—we all want to be happy and live well"* (2013).

This is the premise of this book. Despite any loss clients may be experiencing, you can coach them to find that happiness again. You can guide them through the process and in the meantime, as you process your own loss, you can also embrace happiness in your heart.

Many types of therapies are available to help our clients feel good: cognitive behavioral therapy, positive psychology, spirituality, mindfulness, meditation, and even yoga. Through them, we embrace a more holistic approach to wellness. This inside-out approach is the philosophy of The 11 Principles of Transformation® system. It brings a transformation from the inside out.

I present this book from a professional personal perspective, as I lost my beloved father when I was 12 years old. Because of this loss, I dedicated many years of my adult life to study about the psychology and spirituality of death and dying. I focused on the bereaved and their grieving process, until I realized, after working with so many people facing challenging life transitions, that grief is not only the response to the death of a loved one, but to any loss we experience in life.

With this realization in mind, I wrote the self-help book, *Transform your Loss: Your Guide to Strength and Hope,* and dedicated it to the memory of my father. This book is where I introduced the system, *The 11 Principles of Transformation,* because I wanted to share with people core principles that could help them embrace life again, after a loss. The principles are not original. They are perennial. What is unique is the way the system was conceived; its main purpose is to offer a roadmap to help people transform their loss into personal growth.

I am pleased to present this system, which evolved into *The 11 Principles of Transformation*. I share it in seminars for professionals who work with clients facing a major life transition, and in workshops I facilitate for people who are facing their own losses,. The content presented in this workbook is a compilation of material gathered throughout the years of working with clients—from my books, workshops, and the online program. It touches my heart to see people experiencing breakthroughs in their lives as they are transformed. Therefore my slogan, *Transform Your Loss . . . Transform Your Life.*

At the end of 2014, I started teaching the material for PESI, and a great part of this book is based on those presentations. Now you have a manual filled with suggestions you can use with your clients to help them transform their lives after a loss.

HOW THE BOOK IS CONCEPTUALIZED AND ITS STRATEGIES

The book is divided in two sections: *Understanding Loss and Grief,* where we elaborate on the concept of losses and how grief is manifested, and *The 11 Principles of Transformation.*

Throughout the book you will see the word *strategies.* These are suggestions to be used with your clients, individually or in group activities. You know your clients and know what works best for them.

In the second section, you will find the following three elements that are consistent throughout the principles:

- Meaningful quotes   • Affirmations   • Meditations

These elements are included in all principles as a format to be used as you start and finish each principle. At the beginning you will be directed to do the same type of exercise with your clients utilizing quotes. This will help indicate how they are doing in their process as they advance in their transformation process. I have found them to be extremely valuable to help people express their grief and empower them into their new reality.

I will share with you how I use the principles either individually or in group activities to help people focus on their strengths and embrace life with hope and strength.

The principles can be applied to present and past losses. It can also serve as a guide for dealing with future losses. The purpose is to give clients tools and techniques that can help them in all areas of their lives as they experience losses and challenges on regular basis. The philosophy is to respond instead of react and to know that even if it is true they may have not chosen the event, they can always choose their response.

In life, we have choices. If clients are facing a difficult life transition, they can choose to let go, to stay still, or to remove the pain. It is up to them. What will help them in their transition is acceptance of the situation they are confronting. It may not be easy, but if they face it with inner strength and hope, they will be able to embrace life and find joy again.

Your client may have had one of those moments when the world seems to have stopped and all they feel is void. I felt it when I was 12, when I just wanted the world to stop and stay still. But the world continued moving and I HAD to learn to continue moving with it. It was hard. It was sad. It felt unbearable, but I was able to continue. I was able to transform my loss into growth. Helping your clients to also transform their loss is the purpose behind this book. I offer it to you with all my love and care, with the hope that it will provide you with a roadmap you can share with your clients who are facing a loss in their lives.

PART I

UNDERSTANDING LOSS AND GRIEF

Chapter 1

Become a Transformative Agent in the Lives of Your Clients

As mental health practitioners, we care for our clients and want to be present as they process their grief. Now, what about you? Have you embraced and processed your own story of loss and transformation? If we are in touch with our own losses and have taken the time to process them and transform them, we are better able to be an agent of change for our clients.

Now, it is essential your clients understand that for the system to work (and it does!), they need to do their part. They need to commit to their own transformation. They need to take responsibility for their own well-being and take one step at a time. It may be challenging at the beginning, and you may have resisting clients who may give you excuses for not following through. However, if they are searching for help, it means they have not lost all hope. They want to feel better. The only way your client can achieve an inside-out transformation is by acknowledging the innate power he or she has.

We can be a caring and skilled guide, educator, or therapist. However, if your client does not use his or her inner resources, the healing process will be difficult to achieve. We do not have the power of changing how they feel. This is based on the choices they make and the connection with their inner selves. Therefore, as a healthcare professional, it is extremely helpful for you take into account the thoughts, feelings, and behaviors of your clients as they experience grief. This perspective will provide a more solid foundation and insight to know which technique would help your client the most. In this book, we will cover many techniques. Therefore, the more you know about your client's worldview, the better the results will be in your work with them.

For the past 12 years, I have been an adjunct professor of Death and Dying. I have taught at Florida International University (FIU) and Kaplan University, and this experience has given me the opportunity to realize the need that exists for education in the area of grief and loss. Additionally, as the former grief & growth leader coach of the International Coaching Academy (ICA), I understand the role of coaching when clients want to feel empowered when processing their grief. Many times clients do not know what to expect or how to go about daily living with their grief. We are there to guide, coach, and educate them. It is a transformative process. It is a meaningful relationship.

Chapter 2

Loss: Assessments and Evaluations

What is loss? Is it the same for everyone? Is it possible to grow through loss?

Most of your clients, when talking about facing a loss, may think you are *only* referring to the death of a loved one. As mentioned earlier, the paradigm we use in this book regarding loss is not limited to death, but encompasses a broader view.

Because loss is a subjective process, we need to open our hearts and allow our clients to express their pain and share their loss. Furthermore, loss is a personal experience and to better understand this concept and capture a broad concept, we will start by exploring different definitions of loss.

> *Loss is defined as the real or perceived deprivation of something that is deemed meaningful. A loss can be death related or nondeath related. A loss experience is one in which a return to some aspect of life that we have cherished or valued is no longer possible.* (Winokuer & Harris)

> *To more fully understand the experience of loss, it is helpful to recognize its universality in human life. In a sense, we lose something at each step along life's journey, from the concrete losses of people, places, and objects we have come to cherish, to the more immaterial but equally significant forfeitures of our youth, dreams, ordeals as we confront life's hard "realities."* (Neimeyer)

> *Each loss is unique and has its own meaning to each individual involved. One cannot know how another feels about a particular loss, but we can help and support each other by using what we have learned from our own experience.* (Bishop-Becker)

> *We experience a sense of loss when something or someone that belonged to us and was of great value has been taken from our lives, leaving in their place a void that we are sometimes unable to fill. This emptiness leaves us baffled, stunned, and with doubts about the next steps on our path. Loss is an experience of our own human condition.* (Houben)

AMBIGUOUS LOSS

This particular type of loss is one I find important to validate, because it may not be easily recognized. Pauline Boss, in her seminal book *Ambiguous Loss: Learning to Live with Unresolved Grief (1999),* introduces us to a human experience many of your clients may be facing or have faced in their lives. According to Boss, two types of situations lead to experiencing this kind of loss:

In Type One, there is physical absence and psychological presence. These include situations when a loved one is physically missing or bodily gone. In Type Two, there is physical presence and psychological absence. In this type of ambiguous loss, the person you care about is psychologically absent—that is, emotionally or cognitively missing. (www.ambiguousloss.com)

LOSS OF THE ASSUMPTIVE WORLD

> *"When a negative life event has challenged one's basic assumptions about the world in a way that these assumptions no longer make sense"*
> — Winokuer and Harris

This may be one of the greatest challenges your clients may experience. They want to have the world they know. It is what gives them meaning and purpose. What happens when this world shatters? What happens when things get out of control and our assumptive world is no longer assumptive? How does this alter the life of your clients?

Simply, we experience a sense of loss when someone or something (keep in mind, it can also be *something*) special has been taken from our lives. This experience, this loss, leaves us with a sense of emptiness, of deprivation, and feeling depleted. However, loss is a universal experience. Nobody told us, and nobody told our clients, when we came into this beautiful world that we would not go through pain, that we would not go through losses. Moreover, the breakup or divorce of a client may not compare to the loss and suffering experienced by a bereaved mother. However, one thing we learn in dealing with grief is that it can't be compared. Your client needs to feel his or her loss is validated.

IT CAN'T BE HAPPENING!

What is the most common response when we hear that someone died, got divorced, or lost their job? No, it cannot happen! I can't believe you! Yes, even *grief professionals* can have this response. Although we know the Five Stages of Grief by Dr. Elizabeth Kübler Ross do not necessarily have a certain order, I believe denial is the typical first reaction. Your clients may have this first response, and we will be talking more about that in a subsequent chapter, when we explore acceptance in Principle I.

Denial is a common response because we are used to our reality and do not want any external factor to change it. Our clients do not want painful changes that alter their own level of comfort. However, from childhood on, we learn life experiences that can turn into losses, depending on how we take them (remember, losses are subjective). In this section we will explore the different types of losses that can be experienced at the different stages of development: childhood, adolescence, as adults, and as older adults.

Each stage brings its own changes, transitions, and losses. What is experienced as a loss when we are children is not the same as when we are adults. Therefore we need to open our hearts and change our perspective. If your clients share with you they had an unhappy childhood, you may especially want to do a history of the losses they experienced as children.

❖
ASSESSMENT
• BEFORE MY LOSS, MY WORLD WAS… •

Complete these statements in your own words.

My personal life was:

Sad and dark and Lost.

My social life was:

non existant secluded.

My health was:

fair

My finances were:

non existant

My professional life was:

non existant

❖ ASSESSMENT

· YOUR CONCEPT OF LOSS ·

Write your own definition of loss:

_____

_____

_____

_____

_____

_____

Describe 5 major losses:

1. _Losing my Mom my world ended_

2. _Losing my sister/best friend feel like I cant breath_

3. _Losing my cousin Devin_

4. _Divorcing my ex husband_

5. _Losing my father to suicide_

ASSESSMENT

• COMMON LOSSES •

Check the ones that apply.

In Childhood

___ Death of parents, grandparents, or sibling	___ Having a parent in the military
___ Divorce of parents	✗ Moving (school or neighborhood)
✗ Pet loss	✗ Moving to a different state or country
✗ Loss of a special toy	___ Illness (loss of health), do a history of primary and secondary losses
✗ Loss of innocence	
✗ Loss of friends	___ Bullying
✗ Loss of only child status	✗ Loss of self-esteem
___ Having a parent incarcerated	✗ Loss of security

Other _____

In Adolescence

___ Loss of your first love	___ Having a parent incarcerated or in the military
___ Broken heart, when the girl or boy doesn't pay attention	___ Moving (school or neighborhood)
___ Loss of scholarship	___ Moving to a different state or country
___ Not being admitted to college	___ Leaving home (away to college). This is one life transition that can elicit two different emotions: joy at being independent, and grief at being away from mom's nurture and family connection!
___ Not making a sport's team	
___ Physical issues (being too fat or too skinny)	
___ Death of parents, grandparents, or sibling	
___ Divorce of parents	___ Illness (loss of health)
___ Pet loss	___ Bullying
___ Loss of friends	___ Loss of self-esteem
___ Loss of a friend due to suicide or car/ motorcycle accident (realizing they are not invincible)	___ Loss of security
	___ Loss due to an absent or emotionally unavailable parent.

Other_____

As An Adult

- ___ Loss of a loved one
- ___ Loss of health
- ___ Loss of a job
- ___ Divorce/relationship
- ___ Loss of a pet
- ___ Retirement
- ___ Loss of security
- ___ Loss of homeland
- ___ Moving

- ___ Abandonment
- ___ Abuse
- ___ Loss of a dream
- ___ Loss of new opportunities
- ___ Loss of material possessions
- ___ Loss of hope
- ___ Loss of trust
- ___ Loss of identity (e.g., sandwich generation)
- ___ Aging parents

Other_____

As Older Adults

- ___ Loss of independence
- ___ Loss of health
- ___ Loss of memory
- ___ Loss of a future
- ___ Loss of youth
- ___ Loss of control

- ___ Moving
- ___ Abandonment
- ___ Abuse
- ___ Loss of material possessions
- ___ Loss of hope
- ___ Loss of trust
- ___ Loss of identity
- ___ Aging parents

Other_____

In adulthood we experience different losses that shake our assumptive world. Because this population may be the age group you work with, I want to expand on how these losses affect our well-being. As it was stated, we experience a loss when someone or something we cared for is no longer with us. The greatest loss we may suffer, based on my own experience, is the loss of a loved one. However, because there are different variables that determine the intensity of the loss (e.g., attachment, relationship, history of losses), it is necessary to pay attention to all losses. For example, a client who is going through a divorce may also experience a huge pain. Although many times people are glad they "are finally divorced" from a person they didn't love anymore or who was abusive, other losses may also come along, such as the change of status, financial losses, or loss of trust.

Another instance is a client who loses his or her health. When we lose our health, our life may change. Our lifestyle, our plans, and our hopes all change, and in many cases, we may lose the motivation to continue fighting or even living.

What about the losses experienced by immigrants? Furthermore, a client who loses a job may have a void that includes the loss of a role and having to deal with the financial implications (more about this in the section about multiple losses). These individuals may even lose confidence, sense of security, or the stamina to look for another job. They may think something is wrong with them and may remain stuck in a place of grief. (Adapted from *11 Myths and Realities Regarding Loss, 2012.*)

MULTIPLE LOSSES

Primary Loss—Secondary Loss

We have been talking about individual losses, but many people experience several losses simultaneously or in close proximity and we call them multiple losses. In some cases, it originates with a primary loss, expanding into secondary losses. Let's take for example the loss of a job.

When you construct the history of losses with your client you will be able to identify and explore each of these losses.

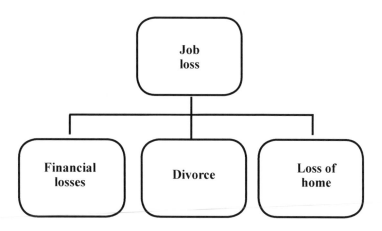

Comparing Losses

Have you ever noticed that when a person is sharing a tragedy (e.g., loss), some people tend to minimize that person's loss or even interrupt so they can say what has happened to *them*? Most people are just waiting to share their story and tell you *their* loss is greater, because in their eyes, it is worse than yours. It is all subjective. It is the loss that happened to them.

As Earl Grollman stated, "What is the worst loss of all? . . . It's when it happens to you or to me. This is our loss" (Kennedy, 2000), and that is the way people feel.

At this point ask your client to share with you the times he or she felt a specific loss was not validated when compared to other losses.

Individual or Group Activities

STRATEGY

· COMPARING LOSS ·

Describe a situation when you felt your loss was minimized when compared to another loss.

How did you feel? What made you feel this way?

What would have made you feel different?

Invalidated Loss

A client may also feel invalidated by statements other people have made. Some of these comments may have been offered with the best intention. However, they may have evoked a sense of invalidation. Some examples are:

- Time heals everything.
- You are so sensitive.
- You are so dramatic.
- You just talk about your loss.
- It's about time you move on.
- Don't play victim.

- You are not the only one suffering a loss.
- Other people have it worse.
- You are lucky *only* this happened.
- But you are doing so great!
- God doesn't give you more than you can handle.

Individual or Group Activities

STRATEGY

• INVALIDATED LOSS •

Ask your client to sit in a comfortable position. You may want to play some soft music in the background, offer a blanket, and assure her she is in a safe place.

Let her know you will be guiding her to connect with her emotions and be able to release them.

Now, take the list of the invalidating statements and read them out loud, taking a pause after each statement. Ask your client to focus on how she feels and to pay attention to any sensation in any part of her body. If it is a disturbing sensation, invite her just take a deep breath and let it go.

Take your time in doing this exercise very slow. You may want to have a box of tissue available.

At the end of this exercise, ask …

• Does this feel especially tender?

• Do you still experience a sense of invalidation when sharing a loss?

• Do you invalidate other people's losses?

HISTORY OF LOSSES PRESENTED IN DIFFERENT FORMATS

In order to have a comprehensive idea of the life experiences of your client, it is a good idea to include a history of losses. I offer it in different formats, so the clients can choose the style that resonates most with them. In doing this exercise, clients revisit life transitions they feel were painful, and you help them identify losses.

Why would our clients be interested in revisiting their losses? Why would they care? Well, besides giving us a broad idea of how their lives have been and what types of losses they have experienced, it will give them the opportunity of discovering their patterns of grieving, their coping skills, and their strengths (and challenges) when dealing with a loss.

STRATEGY

· HISTORY OF LOSSES ·

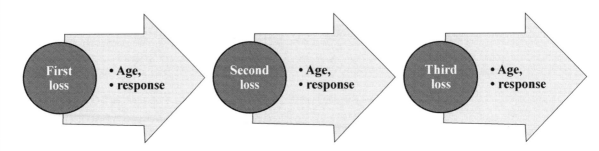

Ask your client to do the following:

Start with the most recent loss, back to the earliest you remember. Remember, a loss is any life transition that causes grief or suffering.

The important thing here is to know your response and the response of your significant others to YOUR response.

Example:

LOSS: Snow White (my rabbit)

AGE: 8 years old

MY RESPONSE: Crying, deep sadness, longing, guilt (not allowing her to have babies)

RESPONSE OF MY SIGNIFICANT OTHERS: My mother tried to calm me down, expressing it was an animal. Now that I remember, she allowed me to wear black and white (based on the customs of that time, mourning was expressed wearing black) for a month. But on my birthday (two weeks after), I had to wear a shocking pink belt, with shoes of the same color.

ASSESSMENT

• HISTORY OF LOSSES •

My first loss was:

_____

_____

_____

_____

At age: _____

My response was:

_____

_____

_____

_____

My family's response was:

_____

_____

_____

_____

These strengths helped me:

_____

_____

_____

_____

I had the following challenges:

_____

_____

_____

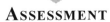

• EVALUATION OF YOUR LOSS •

Please circle the statements you identify with.

1. I do not want to think about my loss.

2. I will never be happy again.

3. These misfortunes only happen to me.

4. Everyone else is happy.

5. I do not care about my health.

6. I do not believe in support groups.

7. I do not believe in God.

8. I do not believe in spiritual guides.

9. I feel a lot of anger.

10. I feel a lot of resentment.

11. I will never forgive those who caused this pain.

12. I do not want to talk about death.

13. Life is unfair.

14. If I get busy, I do not need to think about my loss.

15. I do not have to share my pain with anyone.

16. I need to be strong for others.

17. From now on, I will not show my feelings.

18. I do not think I will recover.

19. Nobody understands me.

20. I will never see my loved one again.

21. Religion does not help to heal a loss.

22. Why did this happen to me?

23. I am guilty of suffering this loss.

24. Someday I will be happy.

25. I will learn to live with this loss.

26. I will get over this loss and transform my life.

27. I would rather be alone.

28. I do not want help.

29. I have processed my loss.

30. I will be happy again.

31. Losses are part of life.

32. Everybody faces tough times in life.

33. Support groups can provide help.

34. I believe in the possibility of something greater than myself.

35. At certain times we need spiritual guides.

36. Keeping grudges is not healthy for my soul.

37. I have managed to forgive.

38. It is necessary to talk about death.

39. Sometimes life is not easy, but I still go forward.

40. Although it is difficult, I need to process my loss.

41. It is important to show my true feelings.

42. There will be a time when I will have recovered.

43. There are people who understand my pain.

44. I always carry my loved one in my heart.

45. The spiritual dimension helps me to find meaning.

46. I am not the only person facing a loss.

47. I am not guilty of this loss.

48. I help others with their loss.

49. I can love, starting with myself.

50. By transforming my loss I can change my life.

ASSESSMENT

• LOSS TIMELINE •

Create a timeline with significant losses and the age at which they occurred, using the following timeline as an example.

EVENT	Birthday	Moved to another school	Parents got divorced	Father died	Lost scholarship	Divorce/job loss
AGE	9	14	15	21	31	32
EVENT						
AGE						
EVENT						
AGE						
EVENT						
AGE						
EVENT						
AGE						
EVENT						
AGE						

Exercise

• IMMIGRATION LOSS •

Please circle the losses you have experienced.

Loss of a loved one

Loss of health

Loss of a job

Divorce/breakup

Loss of homeland

Loss of state (relocating)

Loss of the "assumptive world"
(e.g., what is known to us)

Loss of expression

Loss of identity

Loss of self-esteem

Loss of profession

Loss of language

Loss of friends

Loss of traditions

Loss of family values

Loss of family connectedness

Loss of appropriate care

Loss of hope

Loss of dreams

Which has been your greatest loss living in a new country or state?

_____

_____

What do you miss the most?

_____

_____

What has helped you cope?

_____

_____

What hasn't helped you?

_____

_____

What would have helped you?

_____

_____

Source: Adapted from *Counseling Hispanics Through Loss, Grief and Bereavement:*
A Guide for Mental Health Professionals by Ligia M. Houben (Springer, 2009).

Significant power can come from acknowledging past losses. They all have a meaning in the lives of your clients, so it is important to never minimize them, even if they "feel" or "look" insignificant.

Maybe your client has never had the opportunity to talk about what has happened to him or her, and you provide an opportunity for that client to do so.

Is it helpful to share our story?

If you have a history of loss, it can be meaningful to share with your client a helpful technique or resource that helped you to move forward with hope and strength. If we are in touch with our own losses, and have taken the time to process them and transform them, we can be an agent of change to our clients. When I conduct seminars with clients, I always start with sharing my own losses to put us all on the same level of humanity.

In my life I have gone through my own share of losses. These are some of the most important ones:

- At 12 I lost my father, which has been my greatest loss and for whom my book *Transform Your Loss: Your Guide to Strength and Hope* was written.
- At 13 I lost my home in an earthquake.
- At 19 I got divorced.
- At 20 I moved to the United States. I lost my homeland.
- At 22 I lost my health; I suffered from an eating disorder.
- At 54 I lost my health when I was hit by a car while crossing the street.

FAMILY DYNAMICS WHEN DEALING WITH LOSS

> *The family of origin is the environment that initially shapes our understanding of what "normal" is for us.*
>
> — Linda A. Curran

We know that each family has dynamics on how to behave when facing challenges or losses.

The family of origin greatly influences a person's values, beliefs, and behaviors. Social organization is based on the values and beliefs ingrained in a culture, and they are generally learned from family.

Your client may be used to relying on his or her family system to process grief.

For many of your clients, their family is one of the strongest resources they have in their lives; therefore, knowing the values and dynamics of their family of origin is fundamental to understanding their ways of coping with loss and expressing grief. The following assessments will give you an idea of the dynamic and values of your client's family.

When dealing with losses, your client may already have various coping skills to deal with loss. The following list includes the most common ways to cope. Please ask your client to add her own coping skill, if it is not included here.

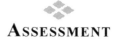

ASSESSMENT

• COPING SKILLS •

	Yes	No
• Abusing alcohol/drugs	_____	_____
• Food	_____	_____
• Sex	_____	_____
• Working	_____	_____
• Shopping	_____	_____
• Ignoring	_____	_____
• Isolation (including computer time)	_____	_____
• Anger	_____	_____
• Fear	_____	_____
• Talking with someone	_____	_____
• Exercise	_____	_____
• Sleeping	_____	_____
• Crying	_____	_____
• Not thinking about it/ignoring	_____	_____
• Sharing with others	_____	_____
• Praying	_____	_____
• Withdrawing	_____	_____
• Social media (e.g., Facebook)	_____	_____
• Family support	_____	_____
• Friends	_____	_____
• Other	_____	_____
• Support group	_____	_____
Live	_____	_____
Virtual	_____	_____
• Aggressiveness	_____	_____
• Detachment	_____	_____

Source: Adapted from *Counseling Hispanics Through Loss, Grief & Bereavement. A Guide to Mental Health Professionals*, 2011.

Individual or Group Activities

STRATEGY

• LIFE COLLAGE •

For creative clients, you can ask them to put together a collage of different life experiences and indicate how they relate to them (this is a great idea as a group activity!). What you need are magazines, images from the Internet (if members of the group are tech-oriented), cardboard, scissors, and glue.

If they want to be even more creative, they (individuals or groups) could also do a PowerPoint presentation to share. This would have to do with the length of the group activity, how many members you have in group, and how comfortable they feel sharing their stories.

The purpose is for your client to elaborate on the impact these losses had on his or her life.

Ask your client the following:

- Have you processed your losses or do you still feel *tender*?
- Did you experience personal growth?
- How has the loss influenced your life?

GROUP STRATEGY

• STORYTELLER •

Choose a role to play. You will have 7 minutes to play each role. So, independently of the role you start with, you will be able to play them all.

Roles: • Storyteller   • Active Listener   • Observer

After the 21 minutes, participants to come together as a group and share their experience.

- How did you feel being the <u>STORYTELLER</u>? Any challenge? Any benefit? What did you learn?

- How did you feel being the <u>ACTIVE LISTENER</u>? Any challenge? Any benefit? What did you learn?

- How did you feel being the <u>OBSERVER</u>? Any challenge? Any benefit? What did you learn?

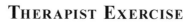

THERAPIST EXERCISE
· YOUR HISTORY OF LOSS ·

As we help clients to be aware of their life experiences, we can also be present to our own lives and elaborate the history of our losses. This reflection will help you get in touch with your inner self, process the losses that may still feel tender to you, and feel authentic when helping your clients process their own losses.

What memory of your life feels tender?

_____

_____

_____

_____

Do you find yourself saying invalidating comments?

_____

_____

_____

_____

What makes you do that?

_____

_____

_____

Would you be authentic working with your client through losses if you have not gone through your own history of losses?

_____

_____

_____

Embrace and process your own story of loss and transformation. If we are in touch with our own losses, and have taken the time to process them and transform them, we can be greater agents of change to our clients.

Chapter 3

Grief: Types, Dimensions, and Manifestations

> *Do not be afraid of pain. It is part of life.*
> *Instead, prepare yourself mentally, emotionally,*
> *and spiritually, when it knocks at your door.*
>
> — Ligia M. Houben

What is grief? How is it experienced? Does everybody express it the same way?

Helping clients understand what grief is, and how it is expressed, can be challenging, because many people assume grief is only expressed by crying. In this chapter we will explore the different types of grief, how it is expressed, and how it differs among individuals. Essentially, grief is the natural and unique response to a loss. I say it is *unique*, because as human beings, we are all unique; therefore our grief is unique. What we need to keep in mind is that each of us has our own story and ways to process grief.

Defining grief can vary when viewed from different perspectives. I have included the following definitions you can share with you clients as quotes, asking which definitions resonate the most with them.

Grief is a global phenomenon and any person who develops the "heart, head, and hands" dimensions of providing care has the potential to become an exquisite witness to the journey of a grieving person. (Jeffreys)

The grief response can be compared to snowflakes, where we can look at the flakes and identify them as "snow," but when you look closer, the crystalline structure of each individual flake is unique, and there are an infinite number of patterns that can be found." (Winokuer & Harris)

The terrible emotional pain of grief tends to have a life and process of its own. Allowing the process to unfold with mindful awareness—a sense of purpose and direction to the pain—may not remove all distress, but it can soften the sharp edge of pain. (Kumar)

Grievers need to work through to the pain of the loss. Grief can be outrageously painful. An impatient culture misreads this task as "to work through the pain of the loss." In other words, to get over it ASAP. (Smith)

Individual or
Group Activities

STRATEGY

• WHAT IS GRIEF? •

Write your own definition of grief:

_____

_____

_____

_____

TYPES OF GRIEF

Anticipatory Grief

Anticipatory grief is produced when we are expecting something to happen that we know will hurt us deeply. The event hasn't happened yet, but we are already suffering from the awareness that we are going to suffer a loss.

Complicated Grief

Complicated grief, also known as CG, is a debilitating and intense grief that interrupts the life of the person experiencing a loss. It interferes with the healing process as the person gets stuck in his or her pain. Denial, distractions, avoidance, and acute grief dominate that person's life.

If you suspect your client may be experiencing CG, extra help may be needed, because as the Center for Complicated Grief observes:

> People with complicated grief usually need treatment. There are different ways to approach treatment, but it's important to find a mental health professional or grief counselor who knows how to recognize complicated grief and how to treat it.

Disenfranchised Grief

According to Kenneth Doka (2002), we experience *disenfranchised grief* when the type of loss is not acknowledged and the griever is not recognized because the loss is not socially validated. Moreover, the mourning is private instead of being public. Among the different losses we may find the loss of a lover (homosexual or heterosexual), the loss of a pet, a colleague, coworker, or friend.

I also want to add here, the loss of homeland, home, state, or the transition of retirement may be considered disenfranchised grief.

STRATEGY

• DISENFRANCHISED GRIEF •

Have you experienced any of these transitions that produced your intense pain?

- Having a loved one diagnosed with a terminal illness
- Confirming an upcoming divorce or breakup
- Receiving a *pink slip* or knowing my place of work was downsizing
- Having problems with my creditors (e.g., mortgage company)
- Knowing I would have to leave my country or state
- Knowing my child was going away to college

TYPES OF GRIEVERS

> *Clearly, patterns are influenced by gender, but not determined by it.*
> — Kenneth J. Doka and Terry L. Martin

It's been said that men and women process their losses differently. Generally, people assume that men are stoic and deal with grief by themselves without showing their feelings. Women, on the other hand, are supposed to be emotional and need the support of others. However, the way people process and express grief is influenced not only by gender, but by other factors such as personality, history of losses, culture, and traditions.

In order to understand different styles of grief, the renowned authors, Kenneth J. Doka and Terry L. Martin (2010), classified these styles as follows: instrumental, intuitive, and a blend of both styles, like a continuum. As you explore these styles take into account gender influences them but does not determine them. Let's explore them:

- **Instrumental grief** has been linked to how men grieve. It has to do with cognition and behavior. This kind of griever focuses more on thoughts and action. They tend to "do" things to express their grief.

- **Intuitive grief** is based on expressing emotions evoked by grief. It focuses on feelings and their expression in an overt manner. Emotions such as sadness can be intense and are expressed by crying. This kind of griever tends to experience grief in an acute and deep way.

- **A blended style** falls somewhere between on this continuum.

TERMS RELATED TO GRIEF

Because the terms *bereavement* and *mourning* are sometimes used as synonymous with *grief*, we will define them, because they do in fact have different meaning.

Bereavement: Bereavement is the period or state of grief and mourning after experiencing the death of a loved one. According to John Wilson (2014), this stage "*is what happens to you.*"

The bereaved feels robbed or dispossessed of someone dear and special to them. This sensation provokes the feeling of void inside of them.

Mourning: Mourning is the outward expression of grief and loss, and it involves physical activities or gestures. For example, when one experiences the death of a loved one, a funeral and/or wake is customary to express mourning. It may also involve wearing a specific color of clothes, engaging in specific activities, or expressing grief through crying, praying, or celebrating dates that hold special meaning. Mourning is highly related to the culture, traditions, and/or religion of the bereaved.

• MOURNING EXPERIENCES •

What are the mourning practices of your culture and/or religion?

_____

_____

_____

_____

_____

Do you feel comfortable expressing your grief in public? How do you express it?

_____

_____

_____

_____

_____

What activities have helped you in your grieving process?

_____

_____

_____

_____

_____

What activities would you like to do because you know they would help you in your process?

_____

_____

_____

_____

_____

MANIFESTATIONS OF GRIEF

When we talk about grief in society, people tend to focus on the emotional aspect (e.g., crying). However, grief can be manifested physically, emotionally, socially, and spiritually. In this section, I want to introduce you to the concept of seeing your client in a holistic manner. We are not only our body, or mind, or spirit. We are a whole person, so the ideal is to work with our clients in a holistic manner. It is good to suggest to clients to get a physical with their doctor to rule out any illness or physical condition.

> *Psychosomatic medicine specifically refers to physical disorders of the mindbody, disorders that may appear to be purely physical, but which have their origin in unconscious emotions.*
>
> — John E. Sarno

ASSESSMENT

• MANIFESTATIONS OF GRIEF •

Consider these common physical, emotional, social, and spiritual manifestations and check the ones that apply.

PHYSICAL   OTHER

___ Headache   ___ Tightness on the chest   _____

___ Stomachache   ___ Lack of appetite   _____

___ Dizziness and nausea ___ Excessive eating   _____

___ Back pain   ___ Lack of sleep (insomnia)   _____

___ Heartache   ___ Too much sleep   _____

EMOTIONAL

___ Depression   ___ Numbness   _____

___ Anxiety   ___ Sadness   _____

___ Fear   ___ Anger   _____

___ Hyperactivity   ___ Guilt   _____

___ Lethargy   ___ Shame   _____

___ Mistrust   ___ Achiness   _____

___ Despair   ___ Remorse   _____

___ Shock   ___ Emptiness   _____

SOCIAL   _____

___ Isolation   ___ Excessive shopping   _____

___ Poor communication ___ Excessive computer use   _____

___ Excessive going out ___ Excessive texting   _____

___ Overwork   _____

SPIRITUAL   _____

___ Lack of faith   ___ Anger toward life   _____

___ Inability to forgive ___ Closeness to church (temple) _____

___ Lack of hope   ___ Closeness to God   _____

___ Anger toward God ___ Finding meaning in the loss   _____

METAPHORS OF GRIEF

Grief is a process. It is not stable or static. One of the best metaphors is that of a rollercoaster. If you have been in a rollercoaster, you know the feeling. It goes up and down and has sudden turns. It is unpredictable and is not linear. Life is not linear. Grief is not linear. It has its ups and downs.

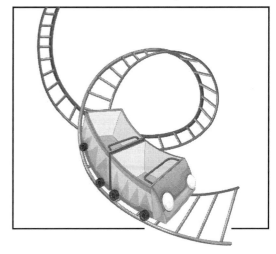

I always use this icon in my presentations so people can identify with the feeling. For example, during one workshop, a man shared that this concept of a grief rollercoaster reminded him when he was a young kid and rode Space Mountain (a rollercoaster in Disney World). He remembered it was dark and that he experienced a *horrendous* fear when he was going *down and down*, which can be compared to times when your client experiences those "dark days." On the other hand, he or she may experience a "high moment," just like when one is on the "top" of the rollercoaster. He or she may think "Oh, I am over this pain." (Remember that society is good at sending us the message to "get over it.")

What happens, then, when pain comes back as a wave? Clients may be confused and lost with their own reaction. This is an important concept to share with clients, so they know that during special occasions such as anniversaries, birthdays, or the holidays, they may have those "low" moments. Many times these moments also happen when listening to a special song, going to a special restaurant, or looking at pictures.

Besides the rollercoaster with its ups and downs, another metaphor I find evocative when we experience grief is that of a tornado. When we are grieving, we feel a devastating sensation inside, comparable to a tornado. For this reason, when I do my seminars, I also use a picture of a tornado to illustrate the intense sensations of pain and destruction. It is a graphic representation of grief to me.

Individual or Group Activities

STRATEGY

· DRAW YOUR GRIEF ROLLERCOASTER ·

Ask clients to draw a rollercoaster, and identify their down and up experiences.

EXERCISE

· TORNADO SENSATIONS ·

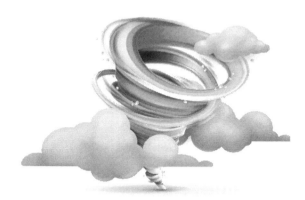

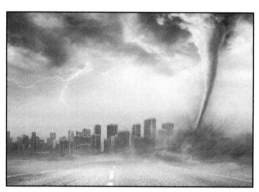

Choose one of the tornado pictures and write about the emotions you are experiencing.

- Scared
- Dark day
- Dynamic
- Chaos

- Storm
- Hope
- Adventure
- Uncertainty

- No escape
- Transformation
- Turmoil

_____

_____

_____

_____

_____

_____

_____

When your clients experience acute grief (just like having the tornado inside), they may tell you, "I cannot continue living without my loved one" or "I will never be happy again."

When they are in that space, what they need the most is your support, your compassion, and your helping hand. At this time, the last thing they want to hear is for them to be strong or that growth will come through this experience (which will hopefully happen eventually, as they embrace the principles). As we explore each principle, and you realize it is a healing and growing process, you will see how this is based on their clock, and how they are processing a particular loss.

Because grief is the expression of how clients feel and how they perceive their loss, their thoughts greatly influences how they feel. In Principle IX (*Modify Your Thoughts*), we will expand on this concept and how clients can be empowered through their own thoughts. Grief can be debilitating and scary, and some people may even feel they are losing control or "going crazy," because of their changing mood swings or their intrusive thoughts. These thoughts may be one of the reasons they have come to see you or join a support group.

> *To spare oneself from grief at all cost can be achieved only*
> *at the price of total detachment, which excludes*
> *the ability to experience happiness.*
>
> — Erich Fromm

STRATEGY

• AM I CRAZY? •

Ask your clients to write down thoughts that have made them think they are "going crazy." Then explore their thoughts and what made them think that way.

CLARIFYING THE STAGES OF GRIEF

When I took my first class on Death & Dying more than 20 years ago, it seems the concept of the stages of grief by Elisabeth Kübler-Ross was different from what it is today. Back then, it was taken as "something" that happened to the grieving person, and it was expected to happen in a linear manner. However, Kübler-Ross explained these could be circular, and with the passing of time, these stages have evolved into a new understanding, taking into consideration the variety of ways people respond to a loss. Moreover, as grief expert David Kessler states, the stages of grief are "part of the framework that makes up our learning to live with the one we lost. They are tools to help us frame and identify what we may be feeling. But they are not stops on some linear timeline in grief. Not everyone goes through all of them or in a prescribed order."

However, because they are so well known and most people experience at least one of these stages, I wanted to include them so your clients can identify them in their own process. These stages have been taken out of context to the point that lay people even tell the bereaved "you are in stage 2 or 3." One of your roles, as a mental health care professional, is to educate your client and help to dispel myths and misunderstandings with the grieving process.

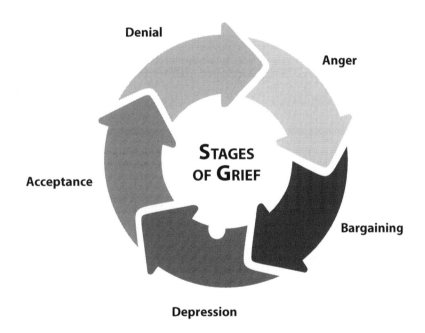

Denial

Denial is a natural reaction when we hear about a loss; it is a way to escape from an unbearable pain. It is our way of protecting ourselves from suffering more than we can handle. Some of the most common responses are: "I can't believe it!" "It can't be true!" "This is a mistake!" "You are wrong!" However, if we suppress our emotions or pretend nothing has happened, we risk behaving in ways that are not healthy, such as abusing alcohol or avoiding talking about the loss. The next questionnaire will give you an idea if your client is having a hard time accepting the situation and is in a place of denial.

STRATEGY

• ARE YOU IN DENIAL? •

Ask your client which of these sentences they are saying to themselves, and then ask them to write down their thoughts and emotions that arise.

It is impossible!

This can't be real!

I do not want to think about what has happened.

Anger

Anger is a common (and many times unacknowledged!) response to a loss. In Principle IV, we will explore different emotions we experience while recognizing our anger and working through it. Anger may happen before the loss happens, or after, or both.

Bargaining

We engage in bargaining when we want to get something and we offer something in return. We say, "If you do . . ., I will do this." We may use bargaining as a way to prevent a loss. We do not want to face the inevitable. We want the situation to get better. Furthermore, if the person is religious, he or she may bargain with God, with promises such as, "If you cure my child, I promise I will start going to church every Sunday."

Depression

After we realize the situation will not change and the loss has happened, we get sad. We grieve over the loss of our loved one, the change suffered in our lives, and wonder how to continue. It is a natural and common stage to go through. Pain is not easy. It hurts. This stage, as with the rest of the stages, doesn't happen in a linear fashion. The person may feel depressed, go back to being angry, deny a loss has happened, and go back to being depressed.

Acceptance

When the person is ready to accept the reality of what has happened to them, they reach this stage. It is the most challenging of stages because, although it doesn't mean you are fine, it happened. You take it as your reality. Let's keep in mind these stages go in a circle, so the bereaved may accept the reality one day, and the next, because of the intense pain he or she experiences, may go back to saying "This is not real."

The answer that clients give to the following exercise will indicate to you whether they are still denying the situation or are ready to accept their new reality.

Exercise
· DENIAL OR ACCEPTANCE ·

Write all your thoughts and ideas for the following questions.

What loss am I experiencing now?

_____

_____

How has my life changed?

_____

_____

What can I do about this change?

_____

_____

Have I stopped asking WHY?

_____

_____

How can I ask WHAT FOR?

_____

_____

What makes it so difficult to accept?

_____

_____

Because in society most people do not know what to say or do when someone faces a loss, they may make comments that upset your client. Attitude toward grief reveals itself through the comments people make when talking about loss. These are some of the most common comments:

- *You are strong! You can rebuild your life again!*
- *You are so lucky you had your mother for such a long time.*
- *Your child is an angel now.*

One of the natural responses your client may have is to minimize his or her feelings or put them aside. I call this *putting them on the shelf.* Sometimes it is "necessary" when the bereaved is facing a situation where he needs to take care of urgent matters, such as a murder, accident, natural disaster, or any other type of loss that may involve demanding tasks. In the case of a divorce, it could involve going to court or getting into a custody battle. In the case of losing a job, all the financial challenges and ways to deal with meeting the family needs are imperative.

In these situations, the grieving process may be suspended, because it is necessary to use all the energy in solving important matters. Grief work demands energy, and your client may feel drained and depleted. One of the most common responses in such situations is to minimize one's feelings or divert the emotion.

EXERCISE

• WHAT HELPS, WHAT HURTS? •

Indicate which of the following phrases have or haven't helped in dealing with your loss.

PHRASES	DOES HELP	DOES NOT HELP
Time heals everything	_____	_____
It's God's will	_____	_____
God has a plan	_____	_____
Your loved one is with God	_____	_____
Life is difficult	_____	_____
He/she wouldn't like to see you like this	_____	_____
Move on	_____	_____
You are strong!	_____	_____
Don't cry!	_____	_____
Have a drink!	_____	_____

STRATEGY

• AVOIDANCE BEHAVIORS •

Ask your client if they are engaging in avoidance behaviors such as:

- Denying their feelings
- Avoiding talking about their situation
- Self-medicating with drugs or alcohol
- Abusing alcohol
- Isolating
- Engaging in compulsive behaviors

ACTIVE GRIEF

Because grief is an active process, it involves some tasks that need to be performed in order to assimilate the loss. It involves more than just waiting for a stage to happen, or allowing time to heal. Doing some grief work involves not ignoring the pain and processing it from the inside out. It is only then that your client can transform loss into a personal and spiritual growth.

STRATEGY

• GRIEF WORK •

Do you know how your client feels about processing their grief? What are your client's expectations? Ask your clients to write a few lines about how he or she feels about doing grief work, answering these questions:

Are you hearing a message of ignoring grief from family and/or friends?

How do others deal with your grief?

Are others ready to deal with your grief? What is their reaction?

- They avoid asking about my loss.
- They avoid looking at me eye to eye.
- They pretend nothing has happened.
- They make jokes to make me laugh.
- They try to distract me (e.g., going out).
- They suggest the use of alcohol (e.g., drink a glass of wine or drink and you'll feel better!).

WHAT IS GRIEF WORK?

Grief work is the processing of grief through expressing the feelings associated with the loss, which can occur on several dimensions: physical, emotional, social, and spiritual (Doka & Martin, 2000). This work helps in the healing process by allowing the person to get in touch with feelings, internalizing and processing them.

A realistic approach helps clients understand where they are in their process. Your clients may feel hurried by loved ones, as people push them to move on. What if they are not ready?

It may be they are a widow or widower, or a divorcee, and are told to start dating again. Clients may be confused and ask you how long does it take to start feeling better. They may want to "jump" over the grief work and start comparing themselves with others. Who is right here? Reassure your clients that they have their own clock (covered in Principle II), and the time to grieve is what feels right for them. Remind them that they do not need to please anybody but themselves.

Stuck on A Painful Image

If your clients complain of having a constant memory in their mind that causes them distress, you can help them change a painful image and therefore, the emotion.

The following NLP technique has proven extremely effective in achieving a positive result.

You can do this exercise with individuals or groups, however with individuals you have the benefit of obtaining greater details of the memory.

Individual or Group Activities

STRATEGY

• MOVING PAST A PAINFUL MEMORY •

Imagine you are in a movie theater sitting on a red-velvet chair.

It is very comfortable and you are by yourself in the theater. In front of you there is the screen with the curtains closed. Suddenly they open and you see a blank screen.

Start playing the film of the memory you have in your mind.

You run it like a movie, from the beginning to end. Then, when you reach the end, you rewind the memory really fast to the beginning of the film. Then, you run the film again, from the beginning to the end. Again, when you reach the end, rewind it faster and faster.

After repeating this exercise four or five times, ask your client what he or she is seeing on the screen.

Another technique similar to this one is to see the image in the screen full color and close up. Then, each time the client plays the film, ask them to push the image farther and farther away, and the colors look dimmer, or faded into black and white. Your client pushes it back and back, to the point that it is just a dot. Then, ask your client how he or she feels. Ask whether the same memory remains in his or her head.

Benchmarks and Timelines

We live in an instant gratification society, where everything seems to be rushed. Your clients may feel rushed in their grieving process when people give them benchmarks, such as:

- After three months, you should have cleaned the closet and gotten rid of all your loved one's belongings.
- After six months, you should be able to travel by yourself.
- After one year, you should be dating.

Ask your clients which "benchmarks" they have gotten from friends and relatives and how they have responded to them.

In grief it is essential to be culturally sensitive because grief is not limited to a particular culture. What makes the difference is their grieving style, which includes how we express our grief. As a mental health professional it is important for you to recognize these differences so you can understand your client better.

Special Dates

As mentioned before, grief may be intensified during specific times—holidays, birthdays, anniversaries, or any special date—making it feel more challenging. We will concentrate here on the holidays and how you can help your clients cope with grief.

Holidays trigger our memories and because of this, your clients may have a feeling of moving backwards or regressing in their grieving process. Holidays are times when we are supposed to be happy, which can make your clients feel overwhelmed, overstressed, and exhausted.

Everyone is expected to show up for the holiday celebration showing their best face, and many times not showing their real feelings, because in our society we are not used to expressing painful emotions during special dates, and it is crucial to acknowledge these emotions.

STRATEGY

• HOLIDAY HELP •

- Have a good support system outside of their family where you can discuss your feelings.
- Prepare a ritual for the celebration to honor your loved one, such as lighting a special candle or placing a box for memories.
- Plan what to say to questions or comments.
- Accept and ask for help in difficult times.
- Consider starting a new tradition.

STRATEGY

· CONNECTING WITH EMOTIONS ·

Ask clients to sit in a comfortable position. You may want to play some soft music in the background, offer a blanket, and assure them they are in a safe place. Let them know you will be guiding them to connect with their emotions and be able to release them.

Now, take the list of the invalidating statements below and read them out loud, taking a pause after each statement. Ask clients to focus on how they feel, to pay attention to any sensation in any part of their body. If it is a disturbing sensation, invite them to just take a deep breath and let it go.

- Time heals everything, so be patient.
- You are so sensitive.
- You are so dramatic.
- You just talk about your loss.
- It's about time you move on.
- Don't play victim.

- You are not the only one suffering a loss.
- Other people have it worse.
- You are lucky *only* this happened.
- But you are doing so great!
- God doesn't give you more than you can handle.

Take your time in doing this exercise. Do it very slowly. You may want to have a box of tissue available, as they may have an emotion stuck in their body.

At the end of this exercise ask them if they want to share in group. As with all meditations, suggest they write in their journal about their experience.

THERAPIST EXERCISE
• PROCESSING YOUR OWN GRIEF •

When exploring the different types of grief and manifestations, have you identified yourself with any of these types of grief and expressions? Do you feel the need to process a past (or present) loss? Remember that in doing your grief work, you allow yourself to release negative emotions that may be manifesting in different areas of your life, including your work.

When your clients share their grief, do you focus on their story, or do you think about your own story?

_____

_____

_____

After learning about the different manifestations of grief, do you feel you are grieving a loss?

_____

_____

_____

How do you express your grief?

_____

_____

_____

Have you ever diverted from grief with alcohol use or any distraction?

_____

_____

_____

Grief is an intense and personal process. Unless we heal from the inside out, we keep the pain deep in our souls. If you realize you have not grieved past or present losses, take this opportunity to do your own grief work.

PART II

From Loss to Growth:
The 11 Principles of Transformation®

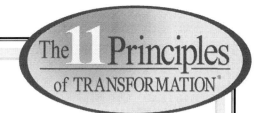

- **Principle I: Accept Your Loss.**
  We will learn how acceptance can be a choice. Your client can choose between dwelling on what has happened or to accepting the new reality and do something about it.

- **Principle II: Live Your Grief.**
  We will learn how to validate the emotions we are experiencing. Your client may be suppressing pain that could be affecting many areas of her or his life.

- **Principle III: Go Deeper into the Spiritual Dimension.**
  Your client will discover the spiritual tools that can make a difference on how to live after a loss.

- **Principle IV: Express Your Feelings.**
  Your client will learn how to connect with his or her inner self and how to express emotions.

- **Principle V: Share with Others.**
  Your client will develop tools to communicate with others in a meaningful way. The better clients can communicate, the easier it is for other people to understand them.

- **Principle VI: Take Care of Yourself.**
  Your client will learn to pay attention to personal needs and develop habits that bring comfort and well-being.

- **Principle VII: Use Rituals.**
  Your client will find out about the value of rituals and learn how to incorporate them into his or her life.

- **Principle VIII: Live the Present.**
  Your client will learn to let go of the past and stop worrying about the future.

- **Principle IX: Modify Your Thoughts.**
  Your client will learn how to change the way he or she feels by changing habits of thought.

- **Principle X: Rebuild Your World.**
  Your client will learn to use inner resources to relocate a loss and realize there is life after the loss.

- **Principle XI: Visualize the Life You Want.**
  Your client will become the architects of his or her own destiny.

Chapter 4

Principle I: Accept Your Loss

> *Acceptance is a choice that comes from the heart.*
> *It is when you decide, either to be a prisoner of the*
> *circumstances or to fly with hope, towards new horizons.*
>
> — Ligia M. Houben

This first principle is likely the most difficult for your clients to embrace. However, it is the foundation for the system to work. If we want to transform a loss, we first need to accept it. Your clients will learn how acceptance can be a choice within their control. Learning this provides them with two types of freedom. One is the freedom from feeling stuck in pain and misery, and the other is freedom to choose a new beginning after a loss. They can choose between dwelling on what has happened or accepting their new reality and doing something about it.

Acceptance is not being glad the loss happened. It is coming to terms with reality; nevertheless, it can be difficult to achieve because the most common reaction to a loss is denial. The first words many of us say when we learn about a loss are "I can't believe it" or "It cannot be happening."

DEFINITIONS OF ACCEPTANCE

Acceptance means minding the core of your problem. Unless you accept it, you cannot solve it. It is like an organic, physiological problem, unless you find it, you cannot treat it. If you cannot accept you have an illness, you cannot heal. It is the same with emotional losses. Acceptance translates into knowing what it is, and then solving it.

It has to do with stopping fighting. If you are going to fight wherever the universe is going to take you it could take you a very long time to get around it. For example, let's think about your clients having panic attacks: unless you realize it is anxiety, and reassure your client he will not die of it, he can't accept it as anxiety. It has to do with going with the flow of what is happening.

I know I have to accept what has happened in order to improve it.

— Definitions shared in seminars or by clients

You need to know where your client is and the concept she has of acceptance. How would you define acceptance? Before working with your client, it is important you know what you understand about acceptance.

This activity can help you know clients' worldview as they give you their own concept of acceptance.

EXERCISE

• ACCEPTANCE •

What does acceptance mean to you?

_____

_____

_____

How can this definition relate to your actual situation?

_____

_____

_____

_____

EXERCISE

• ACCEPT YOUR LOSS •

In this moment, close your eyes and, putting your hand on your heart, reflect on the following questions:

When you hear "Accept your Loss," do you think it is possible? Why or Why not?

_____

_____

_____

What is your reaction?

_____

_____

_____

_____

Meaningful Quotes

> *We cannot change anything until we accept it.*
> *Condemnation does not liberate, it oppresses.*
> — C. G. Jung

> *Acceptance of what has happened is the first step to*
> *overcoming the consequences of any misfortune.*
> — William James

> *Acceptance is not submission; it is acknowledgment of the*
> *facts of a situation. Then deciding what you're going to do about it.*
> — Kathleen Casey Theisen

The use of quotes when working with your client can be an icebreaker. It can be an enlightening and insightful tool that helps the client get in touch with feelings toward her reality. You can use quotes with individual clients, in groups, or even in workshops. You can write quotes on little cards or have them on a list.

As you start working with your client and you want to know where he is in his process of acceptance (because it is a process), you can have quotes in a box or jar and ask him to choose the one that resonates with him the most. This allows him to share with you how he is feeling and how he can apply the quote to his situation.

• MEANINGFUL QUOTES •

What is a meaningful quote for you? Please write it below and then answer the following questions:

_____

_____

_____

What does this quote mean to you?

_____

_____

_____

_____

How can you apply it?

_____

_____

_____

_____

What is important about this quote?

_____

_____

_____

_____

Would you have changed or deleted something from the quote? What? Why?

_____

_____

_____

_____

Individual or
Group Activities

STRATEGY

• QUOTE POWER •

Ask your clients to choose a quote displayed on a table and to sit in a circle.

Ask them to share with the group what made them choose the specific quote. The idea is they apply the quote to their personal situation.

Give them 15 minutes and play some music while they do this activity.

Then, give them a 3 × 5 blank card and ask them to write an empowering quote they feel will help them. Then, ask them to share with the group what made them write those words.

Tell the group to carry this card with them and to read it every day as they wake up. It will remind them of their inner resource to accept their loss. This daily ritual will produce positive changes in their lives.

EMBRACING ACCEPTANCE

As mentioned in the introduction, dialectic behavior therapy is one of the techniques I have incorporated in the 11 Principles, because it can be highly effective in helping people deal with challenging situations. In *Dialectic Behavior Therapy Skills Workbook* (2007), McKay, Woods, and Brandley elaborate on a concept close to Principle I: *Radical Acceptance.*

The authors stress the value of our attitude when dealing with experiences, which will determine how we deal with what has happened to us. They state:

> *By getting angry and thinking that a situation should never have happened, you're missing the point that it did happen and that you have to deal with it. . . . You can't change the past . . . the other option, which radical acceptance suggests, is to acknowledge your present situation, whatever it is, without judging the events.*

Unless we acknowledge our new reality, we can't move forward with our lives. The lack of acceptance keeps your client stuck in a dark place, complaining, dwelling, longing for a different reality, and focusing just on what has happened. It's not that we are happy it happened, but knowing it is the new reality enables moving forward and doing something about it.

What can your client do at the present moment instead of complaining or being angry?

The following exercise is another way you can bring the space to your client to accept their new reality.

EXERCISE

• TELLING THE STORY OF YOUR LOSS •

How did this loss happen?

_____

_____

_____

Who was with you?

_____

_____

_____

How did you find out?

_____

_____

_____

How has this loss affected your life?

_____

_____

_____

What is the hardest part of this loss?

_____

_____

_____

_____

Some people have broken relationships and when they experience a loss, they find ways to get closer to the family, which could show growth. Therefore, despite facing a loss, there has been some gain. Because the purpose is to focus on positive things that may have come out of the loss, ask your clients this open-ended question, so they can elaborate and focus on the positive.

STRATEGY

• FOCUS ON THE POSITIVE •

Despite your loss, have you experienced a positive change in your life? Or some gain?

WRITING THE STORY

If your client has a hard time saying the story in first person, then ask your client to say it in the third person, as if talking about someone else. Then, when the client is ready, the story can be told in the first person. It is a process to move from the third person to the first person. When clients say it in first person, after not being able to accept it, it can be a breakthrough and a validation and owning of their story.

Clients can also describe the story using a metaphor, as in the hero's journey of Joseph Campbell (2008), to transform their loss into growth.

An exercise I frequently do with my clients and have found to be extremely helpful is to write an essay about who they are. This activity will be included in a later principle to enable you to see whether the concept of self remains the same or takes on new proportions or awareness. I have also included a set of question that can be used as prompts or used in addition to writing the essay. You decide what would help your clients the most. I like to have them do both, because it helps them in the process of acceptance.

STRATEGY

• WHO AM I NOW? •

If you are going through a difficult time, how would you feel if I told you "Accept it!" You may resist it and say: I do not want it! Acceptance comes from acknowledging the reality. Ask your client to write a few words on describing "who am I now."

EXERCISE
• YOUR NEW REALITY •

Who are you after experiencing this loss?

_____

_____

How has your life changed?

_____

_____

How have you changed?

_____

_____

What is the hardest aspect of your life to accept?

_____

_____

_____

How would your life be if you accepted it?

_____

_____

_____

How did you feel responding to these questions?

_____

_____

_____

When I am facing a loss my response is:_____

How was this helpful?

_____

_____

_____

What other perspective would help the most?_____

_____

_____

_____

RESTRUCTURE THE ASSUMPTIVE WORLD

William Worden (2009), in his *Four Tasks of Mourning*, talks about the importance of acknowledging the loss and accepting its reality. How can you help your clients restructure their "assumptive world" after a loss? The assumptive world, as we discussed in Chapter 1, is the world your clients know, the one they expect to see every single day when they wake up. What happens when that reality is not there anymore? They may feel someone pulled out the rug from under their feel and their world has shattered. What can you do to help them in that process? You can review what they answered in the original questionnaire (in Chapter 1), and now ask them to answer questions in the "My World Now" worksheet.

As Zig Ziglar says, "It's not what happens to you that determines how far you will go in life; it is how you handle what happens to you." The outcome of this process is based on how your clients will handle what happens to them. And at this moment, they may not know how to go about handling what happened to them, and they are looking for answers and help. You open the space for them to share with you how they *would* like to feel. Maybe at that point it is too difficult to accept their reality or they are unable to make small changes. They may want to continue living in the world they knew and was familiar to them. As their therapist or coach, you do not push them or judge them. You accept where they are and show them new possibilities without disregarding how they feel. Among these possibilities is a reminder of their strengths and how they could use them in this process.

Remind them they have choices in how to respond to the loss, and a strategy that works wonders is to focus on their strengths. The worksheet "Recognizing your Strengths" is a powerful tool to use (page 59).

EXERCISE
• MY WORLD NOW •

After my loss, my world is:

My personal life is:

_____

_____

My social life is:

_____

_____

My health is:

_____

_____

My finances are:

_____

_____

My professional life is:

_____

_____

What can I change of my actual world that is under my control?

_____

_____

How would my world eventually be different if I made this change?

_____

_____

• RECOGNIZE YOUR STRENGTHS •

What does strength mean to you?

_____

_____

_____

_____

What strengths do you have?

1. _____

2. _____

3. _____

4. _____

5. _____

6. _____

How can you utilize your strengths to accept your loss?

_____

_____

_____

_____

_____

_____

_____

_____

_____

_____

EXERCISE ON A ROLE MODEL

The strategy below is based on Neuro Linguistic Programming (NLP) and has proven effective in moments that clients have difficulties in accepting their situation and would like to be able to come to acceptance. Throughout the book I will be sharing with you more NLP techniques, which are especially helpful in empowering your clients.

The basic steps in this exercise are:

- Identify what is difficult for them to accept in their new reality and what they want to be able to accept it.
- Choose a specific context where they would behave in ways that would help them with acceptance.
- Identify a role model: a person behaving the way they wish to behave.
- Encourage your client to engage in the behavior and notice the benefits.

STRATEGY

• ROLE MODEL •

Do you know someone, alive or dead, whom you admire, and who has or had courage and power that you would like to model in working to accept in an active manner what is happening to you?

Do you have someone in your mind you could take as role model who would act in ways you would like to act when it has to do with acceptance and doing something about what is happening to you?

This person could be someone you know or an author, a public figure, just a person that you admire and you would think: *"This person would act this way and I would like to behave like him or her."*

If you do not have a role model, you could imagine your higher self and do the exercise with this image in mind.

Then, share the experience with your therapist or coach and explore the message it sends. It may be like a metaphor. Are you aware of abilities you have that you could apply to their situation?

Individual or
Group Activities

STRATEGY

• HIGHER SELF •

Think about facing a situation that is difficult or painful for you. Then, adopt a bird's eye view and go higher and higher in the air. See yourself at a distance far away from the situation. Try to move higher and higher until the situation looks like a dot. Think about this situation as your Higher Self.

After the exercise, spend some time processing what you felt.

Guide your client through these steps:

Take a deep breath in and now let it out.

Once more, take a deep breath in and now let it out.

Again take a deep breath in and as you exhale slowly, let go of any pain or anxiety, and embrace a calming sensation.

When you are ready, slowly open your eyes.

How do you feel?

EXERCISE

• USING PAST EXPERIENCES •

Think about a time when you thought you would not be able to confront a situation and at the end you were able to do it. Write about it.

What painful situation did you confront in the past that seemed impossible to accept?

_____

_____

_____

What inner resources helped you in your ability to transform your experience?

_____

_____

_____

How can you apply those resources in your present situation?

_____

_____

_____

How do you think you would feel if you allow yourself to be inspired by your past experience?

_____

_____

_____

_____

How would you feel after embracing an accepting attitude?

_____

_____

_____

_____

Because acceptance can be challenging to most people, you want them to feel relaxed and calm. When working with a group, it is a great idea to start the activity with relaxation. You can also start individual sessions with this relaxation technique.

Individual or Group Activities

STRATEGY

• RELAXATION TECHNIQUE •

Time: 5–10 minutes

Technique: Have clients sit on a chair or pillow, or lay down on a mat. Bean bags, which I have in my center and people greatly enjoy, tend to induce relaxation.

Once clients are settled, play soft music, turn the lights low, and ask them to close their eyes. Begin the breathing exercise as follows:

- Take a deep breath counting 1–7.
- Hold that breath for 1–4.
- Then exhale while counting 1–7.

Do this breathing exercise three times, ending with a soft sound of a chime, and ask your clients to open their eyes.

Individual or Group Activities

STRATEGY

• PLAYING MUSIC •

Playing music is also useful in a group setting. Play a song that has to do with acceptance or read a psalm or poem. Then, let clients identify the following:

What memory did the song bring to mind?

What meaning did you find in the lyrics?

With which specific words do you agree?

With which specific words do you disagree?

What made it most difficult?

One of the most healing activities your clients can do is share the story of their loss, because it can be a cathartic experience. In Chapter 1, we covered the history of losses, where they fit on the timeline of all their losses. Now, your clients will focus on saying their stories of loss with the group. They can use the following worksheet as key points to elaborate the story.

If they do not have any present situation that is a loss, ask them to choose one from the history of their losses that still touches their lives.

❖

EXERCISE

• SHARING THE STORY OF YOUR LOSS •

Describe the worst loss you have experienced. You can write it down as a story, with you as the main character.

_____

_____

_____

What made it so difficult?

_____

_____

_____

How did you cope?

_____

_____

_____

Who was present in your life?

_____

_____

_____

ROLE PLAY

Role playing is an activity that can also be cathartic, giving your clients the opportunity to get in touch with their feelings while representing a character. They could come up with a script, as in a real play, or be spontaneous and enact their story. You might also suggest the idea of enacting the different stages of grief, as a guideline of expression.

• YOUR LIFE SCALE •

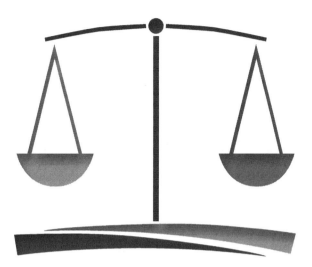

Life is like a scale. The weight goes where we focus. Choose from the following list to help you get a sense of what you are focusing on and where the weight is on your life scale:

- I cannot stop thinking about my loss.
- Things will get better.
- I will never be happy again.
- Nobody understands me.
- Everything bad happens to me.
- I am not able to deal with this pain.
- I am able to confront this transition.
- I am taking care of myself.
- Am I denying what happened to me?

Where is the weight on the scale?

_____

_____

Which actions can I start taking now to change the direction of my life scale?

_____

_____

AFFIRMATIONS

> *Our thinking creates our experiences. . . . Affirmations are positive self-talk.*
> — Louise Hay

Do the following exercise with your clients. Teach them the power of affirmations, because they do have power in how they act in their lives. Invite them to speak the affirmations with hope, conviction, and empowerment.

The affirmations can be said every morning and every night, or whenever needed.

• AFFIRMATIONS •

Now, close your eyes and in your mind, repeat after me the following affirmations. Say these affirmations in an empowered way and make them your reality. You may write them down on a blank card and carry them with you.

- *I am starting a new stage in my life without (the name of your loved one, your homeland, your job).*
- *Loss is a part of life.*
- *I embrace life.*
- *I am able to confront loss.*
- *I accept my reality with an open heart.*

Pay attention to the affirmations. Say, "I am able" so clients are reminded they have the resources. Maybe they are not using them because of their pain; their souls are too bruised. You are there to remind them of transforming a challenge into a possibility.

One of the most important things that can happen is for clients feel they are able to confront their loss, because it provides hope.

For this transformation to happen, it is essential your clients know and feel that they are able to do it. At the beginning, it is common for them to feel unable to accept the loss. However, if they give themselves the message they can do it, their brain starts accepting the new message. When I start working with them or doing seminars, I tell them, "It may not be easy but it's possible," and it is essential to validate their feelings.

Acceptance is a challenge for most people because they assume it demonstrates compliance. However, once they understand its real meaning and the value it has in their transformative process, they will be able to bounce back and take control of their lives with more meaning and empowerment.

MEDITATION

You could also do this exercise as visualization, in a soothing and loving way. You do it slowly and *go with your clients*, so they feel you are with them. You could even record yourself and give them a copy or send it to their email as an MP3, so they can do it at home. Like Dr. Alan Wolfelt says, the most important thing to do is to accompany your clients in their process.

Play soft music and prepare yourself to also be relaxed. Remember, it always starts with you.

• MEDITATION •

Find a comfortable position and very slowly close your eyes. Take a deep breath in and let it go. Take another deep breath and let it go. One more time, take a deep breath and let it go. Now, in your mind, repeat after me:

By confronting my loss and accepting that I am starting a new stage in my life, I have been able to acknowledge that I have the capacity to continue loving and to transform my life. I understand that I have painful memories and moments of doubt; however, I am able to confront them. I embrace them and make them mine. They are a part of the process of accepting this new dimension in my life. I have realized that I suffer such pain because I have a great ability to love and feel.

THERAPIST EXERCISE
• ACCEPTING YOUR REALITY •

As human beings, we all experience loss. When working with our clients, it may feel easier to help them accept their loss than it is to accept our own. It's been said it is easier to help others than ourselves. As you start the transformation process with your clients, embark on your own process. If you have experienced a loss that you found challenging to accept, this is your opportunity to embrace your own transformation. Instead of living by "Do as I say, not as I do," be authentic and transform your own loss.

When you hear the expression, "accept your loss," what comes to mind?

_____

_____

_____

_____

Have you experienced a loss that is a challenge to accept?

_____

_____

_____

_____

What makes it difficult to accept?

_____

_____

_____

_____

What can you start doing NOW to accept it?

_____

_____

_____

_____

Chapter 5

Principle II: Live Your Grief

> *Do not be afraid of pain. It is part of life. Instead, prepare yourself spiritually and mentally when it knocks at your door.*
>
> — Ligia M. Houben

Grief is a unique process and cannot be avoided. It is different for each person because each person is unique. It is necessary to acknowledge it, so we can release it, allowing us to be healed and transformed in the process. Once clients acknowledge their loss instead of denying it, they can continue with the transformation process. Because if they deny a loss happened, how can they process their grief? As we know, grief is the natural response to a loss.

Your clients experience so much pain because they have a great capacity to experience love and feelings.

DEFINITIONS OF THE GRIEVING PROCESS

I thought the grieving process had to do only with the death of loved ones, but as I face my divorce, I find myself experiencing the greatest pain I've experienced. My counselor told me I was grieving.

I never thought my backache had to do with my grief. Now, I understand it can also be physically manifested.

There was a moment in my grieving process when I realized I couldn't continue feeling sorry for myself. It was at that moment when I decided to confront my pain. It was difficult but I was able to work through my grief.

— Definitions shared in seminars or by clients

How do your clients feel about living with their grief? Grief is an emotion and is based on their perception. Have you asked clients how they define **GRIEF**? Their definition will allow you understand their perspective.

EXERCISE

• DEFINING YOUR GRIEF •

Grief is:

_____

_____

You can be creative. If you want, do it as an acronym.

G _____

_____

R _____

_____

I _____

_____

E _____

_____

F _____

_____

When you think about your grief, where do you find yourself in the world?

_____

_____

Describe how you are better processing your grief.

_____

_____

Meaningful Quotes

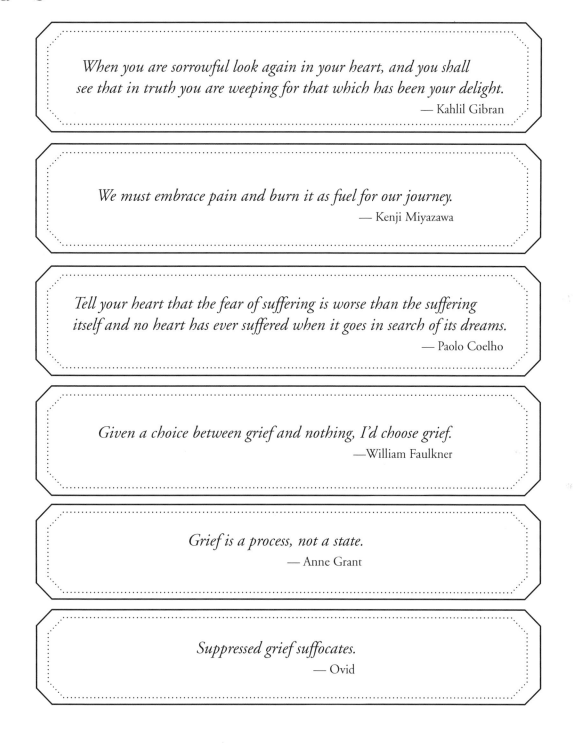

*When you are sorrowful look again in your heart, and you shall
see that in truth you are weeping for that which has been your delight.*
— Kahlil Gibran

We must embrace pain and burn it as fuel for our journey.
— Kenji Miyazawa

*Tell your heart that the fear of suffering is worse than the suffering
itself and no heart has ever suffered when it goes in search of its dreams.*
— Paolo Coelho

Given a choice between grief and nothing, I'd choose grief.
—William Faulkner

Grief is a process, not a state.
— Anne Grant

Suppressed grief suffocates.
— Ovid

As you start working with your clients, the first discovery you want to make is where they are in their grieving process. You can have quotes in a box or jar and ask them to choose the one that resonates with them the most. This allows them to share with you how they are feeling and how they can apply the quote to their situation. You can also provide the following worksheet for homework.

EXERCISE

• MEANINGFUL QUOTES •

What is a meaningful quote for you? Please write it below and then answer the following questions:

_____

_____

_____

What does this quote mean to you?

_____

_____

_____

_____

How can you apply it?

_____

_____

_____

_____

What is important about this quote?

_____

_____

_____

_____

Would you have changed or deleted something from the quote? What? Why?

_____

_____

_____

_____

MAJOR DECISIONS

In our daily lives, we encounter many decisions we must make. Some decisions are easy, others are more difficult. When we are grieving, if possible, it is better to hold off making major decisions. Ask your clients to evaluate any decision they need to make and whether it is easy or difficult. They can always express with you how they feel about those decisions.

STRATEGY

IT'S OK TO LAUGH

One of the greatest questions some of my bereaved clients have is whether it's ok to laugh. Allow yourself some sense of humor. Watch a comedy and give yourself permission to laugh. Because it is easier to focus on other things than embrace grief, your client may divert in different ways. Ask them to answer the following questions:
How do you find yourself diverting from grief?

_____ Shopping   _____ Overeating

_____ Drinking   _____ Overworking

_____ Taking pills   _____ Traveling in excess

When you work with grieving clients, you discover how difficult it is for most of them to "be with their grief." Distracting themselves is like putting a Band-Aid on the wound, hoping it will heal by itself. Our clients could be, for example, going out all the time or overworking.

Clients may be avoiding loneliness at home, wanting to have free time to themselves, or fearing things that trigger their grief. If they live by themselves they do not want to go back to an empty house, so they prefer to divert. When they overwork, after some time, they crash. They get busy and sometimes put their grief process on a shelf. Once all their work is done, suddenly all that stress and fear just lands back on their shoulders. They thought they were done grieving, but they had not gotten there yet, and because they did not really process the grief, it catches up with them. For this reason, the most important thing to do is to process the grief first, because we cannot avoid it.

BEING MINDFUL OF GRIEF

Sameet M. Kumar, in his book *Grieving Mindfully* (2005), applies the Buddhist concept of mindfulness to processing grief in ways that promote awareness and growth. Being mindful means to be aware and conscious of what we experience at the moment (read more about mindfulness in Principle VIII: Live the Now). Here I want to share the concept applied to grief and how you can help clients stop ignoring their grief so they can eventually release it.

Grieving mindfully can be understood as being consciously aware of the intense pain of love after loss. . . . Awareness is not the same as indulging in the intensity of grief. . . . Awareness is allowing yourself to accept the pain of grief, thereby finding relief in not running away from your loss. (Kumar)

DIMENSIONS OF THE HUMAN BEING AND MANIFESTATIONS OF GRIEF

Because I believe that as human beings we have different, interconnected dimensions, I like my clients to approach their grieving process in a holistic manner. In this section, we'll revisit the concept of how grief is expressed in a multidimensional way and give your clients the necessary tools to heal in each of those dimensions.

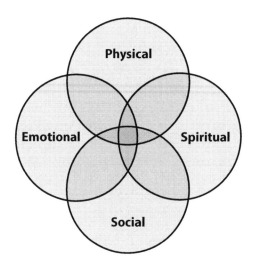

When working with clients, it is good to have a list of manifestations of grief and to ask them which manifestations apply to them. Maybe they do not know they are grieving, and this activity can bring them awareness as they realize grief is manifested in different manners. An important step in the process is to encourage clients to have a physical exam with their doctor, so they know their symptoms are not related to any disease or physical condition.

Your clients may be experiencing backaches, headaches, migraines, stomachaches, dizziness and nausea, among other physical expressions. Our back is a place in our body where many people store pain, grief, or another debilitating emotion, such as stress. When I wrote the self-help book, *Transform Your Loss: Your Guide to Strength and Hope*, I included a story of a young man who developed a backache after the loss of his sister. He never knew his pain was due to unresolved grief, until he had some bodywork done (in Principle VI). What does this incident teach us? That unprocessed grief may get stuck and in many cases expressed through our body.

Heartache is also a common expression of grief and stress. If your client shares with you they have pain in their heart, you have the opportunity to do an exercise known as *Felt Sense*, a term coined by Eugene Gendlin, PhD. It asks your client to connect with how they are feeling in a nonjudgmental and deep manner. The following is a script from Dr. Gendlin.

REFLECTION

• FELT SENSE •

1. **Clear a space.**

    How are you? What's between you and feeling fine?

    Don't answer; let what comes in your body do the answering.

    Don't go into anything.

    Greet each concern that comes. Put each aside for a while, next to you.

    Except for that, are you fine?

2. **Felt sense.**

    Pick one problem to focus on.

    Don't go into the problem.

    What do you sense in your body when you sense the whole of that problem?

    Sense all of that, the sense of the whole thing, the murky discomfort or the unclear body-sense of it.

3. **Get a handle.**

    What is the quality of the felt sense?

    What one word, phrase, or image comes out of this felt sense?

    What quality word would fit it best?

4. **Resonate.**

    Go back and forth between word (or image) and the felt sense.

    Is that right?

    If they match, have the sensation of matching several times.

    If the felt sense changes, follow it with your attention.

    When you get a perfect match, the words (images) being just right for this feeling, let yourself feel that for a minute.

5. **Ask.**

    What is it, about the whole problem, that makes me so _____?

    When stuck, ask questions:

    What is the worst of this feeling?

    What's really so bad about this?

    What does it need?

    What should happen?

    Don't answer; wait for the feeling to stir and give you an answer.

    What would it feel like if it was all OK?

    Let the body answer.

    What is in the way of that?

6. **Receive.**

    Welcome what came. Be glad it spoke.

    It is only one step on this problem, not the last.

    Now that you know where it is, you can leave it and come back to it later.

    Protect it from critical voices that interrupt.

    Does your body want another round of focusing, or is this a good stopping place?

    Eugene Gendlin, Ph.D.

*Reprinted with permission, www.focusing.org/short_gendlin.html.

It is essential your clients get in touch with their emotions because it is not uncommon for bereaved people to feel pain in their hearts and think they are having a heart attack when they are grieving.

Because a client's grief is unique, you may see some of your clients suffer from lack of appetite; others indulge in excessive eating. We know food may be comforting and when eating in excess, the client may be trying to fill up the void he or she feels because of a loss.

A pair of siblings who had lost their mother attended one of my seminars. The sister had gained 20 pounds, and slept all day long. The brother couldn't eat, and had a huge challenge sleeping. Differences are evident, even among family members.

Lack of sleep or oversleeping is another common expression of grief. Sleeping too much provides escape. They may not want to face the reality they are facing. Some clients may tell you they do not even want to take off their pajamas. They may say, "I cannot leave my bed." The good thing is that they were able to leave their bed because they are there with you. In the following exercises your clients will have the opportunity to write down how they are expressing their grief in the dimensions of the human being.

EXERCISE

• DIMENSIONS OF GRIEF •

Express grief related to your four dimensions.

Physical:

_____

Emotional:

_____

Social:

_____

Spiritual:

_____

STRATEGY

• THE GRIEF CLOCK •

Each of your clients has an internal clock.

Ask your client: Is your clock fast? Slow?

Are there times when you hear an alarm? When?

Prompts* that can help them find their own clock include:

When I think about _____ …

I feel? • I avoid? • I embrace?

* A time that can be especially challenging for bereaved clients is when they think, "I can't wait to share this great news with _____." And suddenly reality hits them in the face and they remember that person is not there anymore.

BEING COMPASSIONATE

Compassion starts with us. Your clients need to understand that the grieving process is difficult and unstable. Most of us can be understanding and compassionate with others, but we can be our own worst judge. We expect to think, feel, and behave in an expected manner. If we do not, we get upset, disappointed, and discouraged. Your clients may experience any of these feelings if they believe they are not advancing in their grieving process, often because they expect the process to be linear. Remind them that it takes time and it is not usually a smooth process.

Clients will encounter difficult times, and it is during those moments that they need to be more compassionate, pause, process, and remain hopeful for a brighter tomorrow. It all starts with them.

STRATEGY

• COMPASSION •

Are you compassionate with someone who is grieving?

What about with yourself?

What do you do when you feel so much pain?

BE AN ARTIST FOR A DAY

Expression in art can be valuable and special for your clients. It is helpful to analyze the meaning behind what they create and how they can apply it to their lives. These drawings can be amazingly creative; all of them can be artists. Encourage them to allow emotions to flow on paper or canvas and share the result with others. Ask them to share what was easier to draw: the grief picture or the happy emotion.

For some of your clients, drawing their grief can be especially cathartic.

For this exercise, many clients will draw rainbows and/or sunshine. Another insightful element some people draw is roots, which they may identify with growth or with being grounded. Remind them they don't need to be an artist; they just need to share. Even if they think they cannot feel that way at the present moment, they can always focus on how they want to feel.

• How Do You See Your Grief? •

Today you will use your creative talents to draw what your heart carries inside. You only need to be guided by your feelings. There is no need for talent (if you have it, this is your opportunity to use it!). You only want to have a graphic representation of your emotions; think about when you were a kid and liked to draw or color. This is your opportunity to express what you have inside.

In this box, draw a picture of your grief.

Here, draw the emotion you would like to experience more often.

ART THERAPY

Expressing our feelings through art can be healing. A coloring book for adults is called Therapy in Color™, which you could recommend to clients; or if you are doing a workshop, include it as a group activity.

Invite your clients to allow their grief be expressed in unexpected ways beyond drawing, such as through painting, sculpting, or even dancing!

I worked with a woman who was a ballerina as a young girl. She was very relaxed in doing her work during guided meditation. One day as we were talking about her father, she became emotional and started expressing how much she missed her father. I asked her to find a way to express how she was feeling and to connect with her father. She said her father loved to see her dancing ballet. When I asked her if she thought she could do some ballet movements in the room, she started dancing with her eyes closed and connected with her father in a wonderfully spiritual way.

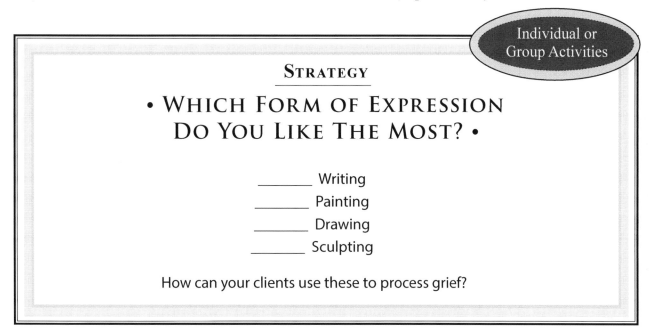

Individual or Group Activities

STRATEGY

• WHICH FORM OF EXPRESSION DO YOU LIKE THE MOST? •

_____ Writing

_____ Painting

_____ Drawing

_____ Sculpting

How can your clients use these to process grief?

Our grief can be experienced in cycles just like the seasons. In the following reflection clients can explore with which season they identify with, depending on their mood and response.

EXERCISE

• SEASONS OF GRIEVING •

When we experience grief, we experience many moods that can resemble the seasons of life. If you like, draw the seasons you are experiencing on a separate piece of paper.

Spring brings a sense of renewal. I feel like this when . . .

_____

_____

_____

Summer is a time when I feel the warm breeze. I feel like this when . . .

_____

_____

_____

Fall is the time when leaves change their color. I feel like this when . . .

_____

_____

_____

Winter is the time I feel the coldest in my heart. I feel like this when . . .

_____

_____

_____

Today I feel _____ because _____.

What is the most prevalent season now? _____

What is my favorite season?_____

ME-TIME

Something we all need, from time to time, is to have a moment with ourselves. In time of grief, this time is precious. I am not implying that being isolated is the goal, but rather to be connected with oneself.

❖❖

EXERCISE

• GIVE YOURSELF "ME" TIME •

Find a private place in your house where you can connect with your inner self and have some me-time. What would you like to do in your special place? Check all that apply.

_____ Write in your journal.

_____ Cry.

_____ See memories of your loved one.

_____ Write letters.

_____ Listen to music that helps you connect.

_____ Meditate.

_____ Just stay still.

_____ Repeat helpful affirmations.

When working with bereaved clients, remind them that love is not restricted by time. I do not believe in telling bereaved clients how long they will be grieving. Losses stay in our heart forever, because love is eternal. The idea is to help clients embrace the love they feel in their heart.

We are going beyond grief. We are taking our clients to a new dimension of hope, joy, and empowerment. Being strong does not mean they cannot cry.

The purpose is to instill in their lives HOPE. Desmond Tutu reminded us that hope is not ignoring the pain, but feeling the ability of embrace life again. This sense is what will inspire your clients to look forward to a brighter future. The following exercise asks clients to describe hope.

> *HOPE is being able to see that there is LIGHT despite of all the darkness.*
> — Ligia M. Houben

EXERCISE

• HOW DO I VIEW HOPE? •

Hope is:

_____

_____

_____

_____

_____

_____

_____

_____

_____

_____

_____

_____

_____

_____

_____

Another way to look at HOPE is:

H _____

_____

O _____

_____

P _____

_____

E _____

_____

CREATIVE STRATEGIES

> *Often the hands will solve a mystery that the intellect has struggled with in vain.*
>
> — C. G. Jung

Sometimes clients may have challenges expressing what they feel. They may even tell you they cannot find words to describe what they are experiencing. Their pain may be too intense.

In such times, using different media of expression can bring them the opportunity to connect with their feelings in a creative way. Art, music, and dance therapy have been used to express to the outer world what is happening in the inner world of the client. It is a way of bringing the unconscious to the conscious.

A Healing Space

If possible, you may want to have a corner in your practice for people to get in touch with their feelings in ways that go beyond words. This soothing space may include inviting furniture, incense, and soft music, whatever helps clients find peace and healing. The purpose of working with our clients during painful moments is to help them find solace when they come to us, and to help them feel better when they leave.

Sandplay Therapy

Originally, sandplay therapy was created to be used with children, but now it *"is rapidly becoming a tool also utilized with adults, couples, families, and groups for healing"* (Labovitz, Boik, & Goodwin, XVI).

The beauty of sandplay therapy is the use of miniature objects to create stories. Clients are able to create their story, sometimes altering the reality and empowering them in the process of playing.

A Sandtray

With a sandtray, clients can play with the miniature figurines, re-creating the story or creating a new one, or just playing with the sand in their hands. For this exercise, play soft music, and leave your client by themselves, so they can connect with their feelings.

This activity can help them express their grief. Then, go back and ask them to share with you any memory, any thought they had, and how they felt. Ideally this technique could be used after you know the story of your client, after having established the connection with them. Furthermore, if they have shared a special song with you, you may play it so they can experience and release it.

There are different types of sandplay therapy, including sandtray or a sandplay box. The store, Brookstone, sells the tray and also the kinetic sand.

Plato's Cave

This allegory of Plato reminds me of grief. It's about people chained in a cave unable to move looking at the shadows of the objects that pass behind them in front of a fire. They think the shadows are the real objects. This is just like grief, if it not processed, people may feel stuck in a dark place. People may stay in a cave, turning their back to the opening. Because they are chained with their own grief, they cannot see the opening behind them or the real object. They do not realize another reality exists. They are just looking in front of them at the shadows of the objects. People are chained and cannot move. It is like clients who are prisoners of what they are feeling. But if you help them release themselves from the grieving chains, they can turn around and see the opening. They can see opportunities waiting for them if they give themselves a chance. They can embrace life again.

You can use this metaphor with your client, and ask them what they think about it. With encouragement, clients can find the relationship of being a prisoner in the cave with their own process of grief. Once they do their grief work, they can let go of the chains that keep them prisoners.

Individual or Group Activities

STRATEGY

• THE POWER OF FOCUS •

Invite clients to notice everything that is white in the room.

Then ask them to close their eyes and then tell you what is blue (you can change the colors, based on the objects present).

Clients will be surprised how difficult it is to recall what is blue, because they had focused on what was white. Then, ask them what this exercise reveals to them.

What is revealed is that reality is what we focus on! Clients whose filter is just grief may be missing beautiful things and the people they still have in their lives.

WHAT WORDS HELP YOUR CLIENT?

People in general, do not know how to deal with grief; therefore they do not know how to express their condolences and may say empty or hurtful words.

One of the greatest complains I hear from clients is that they do not like to hear "I am sorry." Another expression they dislike is, "I know how you feel." People may mean well, but no one knows how we feel. Sometimes your client may not even know how they feel.

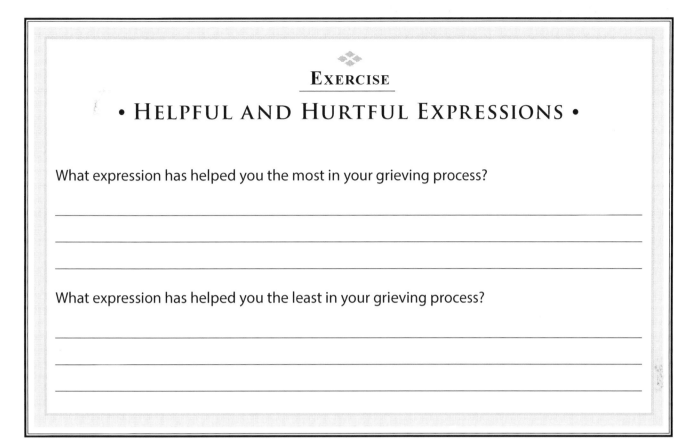

PREPARATION THROUGH EDUCATION

Many people expect grief to better or lessened with time. Your clients may expect that after the second year, they will start feeling better. However, grief cannot be predicted or avoided.

Remind them that grief is not linear, that is often felt like a rollercoaster and manifested in different ways. Give them ideas to prepare themselves for special days, strategies that could help them, including writing in a journal how they feel so they keep track of their emotions. Other grieving triggers can be special songs, special places (restaurants or stores), clothes, poems, movies, cards, stories, and pictures.

Furthermore, on some dates, grief "feels" more intense, including anniversaries, birthdays, Mother's Day or Father's Day, to name a few. At these times, when your client is supposed to celebrate, celebration is difficult and grief is intensified because of the absence. Especially at the holidays, as mentioned in Chapter 2, we are supposed to be joyful, to be in the "spirit." The family may expect the bereaved to be happy and celebrate. At these times communication is especially valuable. Teach clients how to communicate what they expect from others. We will expand more on this topic in Principle V.

Experiencing a major transition or loss brings pain and often a sense of hopelessness in the lives of clients. In this pain and hopelessness, many ask "Why?" It may be more helpful to encourage them to ask "What for?" rather than "Why?" In subsequent principles (VIII–X), particularly in Principle X, we will expand on the value of shifting the perspective of the loss your client is suffering toward being able to find meaning in his or her grief.

• AFFIRMATIONS •

Affirmations can be said every morning and every night or whenever a grieving person needs a reminder.

Now, close your eyes and, in your mind, repeat after me the following affirmations in an empowered way and make them your reality.

- *I can get in touch with my pain.*
- *I choose to let go of the pain.*
- *I know my pain is not forever.*
- *I dedicate sometime each day to feeling my grief mindfully.*

You may write them down on a blank card and carry them with you.

• MEDITATION •

Always remember to set the environment for meditation, with soft music, candles, incense, and oil on hand. If you wish, you may rub some lavender oil in your hands and bring one hand close to your client's nose as they inhale. This would give them a sense of calmness. Before doing this, make sure they are not allergic to lavender or any other oil.

Find a comfortable position and very slowly close your eyes. Take a deep breath in and let it go. Again take another deep breath and let it go. One more time, take a deep breath and let it go. Now, in your mind, repeat after me.

The transformation process requires confronting my pain, not avoiding it. In the moments that I feel pain in the depths of my soul, I will receive and embrace my pain. It is part of me. Each day, I will take a moment to write about what I feel and why I am feeling that way. If I need to cry, I will, because little by little, I will start to feel better. I will become stronger and my life will take on more meaning.

THERAPIST EXERCISE

• PROCESSING YOUR OWN GRIEF •

In this principle, we have explored ways your client can get in touch with their grief and express it in a healing manner. If you find yourself grieving over a loss you were never able to embrace and then, release, this may be your opportunity to do it. Open your heart to the experience and be ready to live your grief.

After exploring the different definitions of grief, is there one that resonated with you?

_____

_____

_____

_____

Have you ever expressed grief in an artistic way? How? If not, which medium touches your heart the most?

_____

_____

_____

_____

What are some of the manifestations of grief you can personally identify with?

_____

_____

_____

Do you find it difficult to process your grief? If so, what makes it so difficult?

_____

_____

_____

_____

Chapter 6

Principle III: Go Deeper Into the Spiritual Dimension

> *When we realize we are pure light and embrace spirituality in our inner selves, our lives begin to unfold in miraculous ways.*
>
> — Ligia M. Houben

In this principle, your clients will have the chance to cultivate spiritual tools that can make a difference in their grieving process. These tools have the potential to be the bridge from a life of complaints and sorrow, to a life of light. It all starts with changing their lives from the inside out.

Gandhi said in his famous words, "Be the change you wish to see in the world."

As your clients embrace these tools, they will be able to be that change in their lives and in the lives of others.

DEFINITIONS OF SPIRITUALITY

I never thought being spiritual was so important. I had lived my life always on the fast track. As I confronted this loss, suddenly I had to stop and reflect. I had to ask myself if I wanted to continue living in a rush all the time, or if I wanted to invite my spiritual self. I am glad I chose to discover my spirituality, which is just to live paying attention and being grateful.

I always thought spirituality was the same as religion, now I know it is different. I can transcend myself and connect with others at a deeper level, with more love and acceptance. To me, this is spirituality.

Spirituality is letting go of unnecessary ties. It's living more freely. It's about forgiving and letting go of the past.

— Definitions shared in seminars or by clients

Meaningful Quotes

The majority of men live without being thoroughly conscious that they are spiritual beings.

— Søren Kierkegaard

Most of us know how important it is to exercise our bodies,
but how often do we exercise our souls?

— Dr. Bernie S. Siegel

We are not human beings having a spiritual experience.
We are spiritual beings having a human experience.

— Pierre Teilhard de Chardin

❖

EXERCISE

• MEANINGFUL QUOTES •

What is a meaningful quote for you? Please write it below and then answer the following questions:

_____

_____

What does this quote mean to you?

_____

_____

How can you apply it?

_____

_____

What is important about this quote?

_____

_____

Would you have changed or deleted something from the quote? What? Why?

_____

_____

STRATEGY

• SPIRITUALITY •

If you want to know how your clients feel regarding spirituality and what practice would resonate with them the most, it is crucial you know their concept of spirituality.

The activity can be done in a setting that invites relaxation. You can dim the light and have some candles. It is an opportunity to connect with that dimension that at times is ignored.

Allow them to share with you their concept of SPIRITUALITY.

SPIRITUALITY OR RELIGION

When I taught a class on World Religions at a local college in Miami, Florida, my students often get these two concepts confused. They asked, "Is there is a difference between religion and spirituality?" The basic difference is that religion encompasses participation in religious activities (pertinent to the organization); there is a personal meaning of religion and private devotional activities within the home. Furthermore, a number of other elements are present in most religions, such as symbols, liturgy, and scriptures, as well as rituals that are observed in public or private worship. According to Harold Koenig, MD (2004), a well-known expert in the field of religion and health, "Religion is a component of spirituality, and one can be spiritual but not religious." And yes, your client can be very spiritual. Some people choose not to follow a religious denomination and yet are still spiritual.

I chose to use the word *spiritual* instead *religion* because I want to be inclusive. If your clients are religious, it is wonderful to incorporate their beliefs, which often help us in facing and confronting pain. Some clients may have a strong faith that helps them deal with their grief. Other clients may not rely on their faith or religion. They may hear from people that if they have faith, they shouldn't grieve. They may feel confused or even guilty. However, a person can be extremely spiritual and not be religious. What matters most is that your clients feel able to recognize their feelings and beliefs, and share them with you. Provide them with a safe place where they realize that as important as it is to have faith, it is important to acknowledge their grief.

I developed a Spiritual Inventory that clients can fill out during this first assessment. The information gained from this questionnaire can give the counselor insight into a client's spiritual beliefs. It was introduced in a manual, *Spirituality and Aging: The Fourth Dimension.* I have used it widely with my clients and in workshops.

You can give your clients a copy of this inventory so they can do it at home. Ask them to bring it back the next time they see you. Just by reading their response to the first question, "Do you have any spiritual needs?" will give you a light on where they find themselves spiritually.

You can also use this activity in group sessions. I suggest playing some soft music and giving the group 15 minutes to reflect. Afterward, they can share with the group the phrases that touched their hearts. Because this exercise is highly profound, I always suggest they elaborate more on their answers when they get home.

❖
EXERCISE

• SPIRITUAL INVENTORY •

- Do you have any spiritual needs?

- Do you believe in a Higher Power/God?

- Where do you find connectedness?

- Do you feel connected to others?

- Do you believe we have a soul?

- How important is forgiveness to you?

- What brings you hope?

- Do you engage into a religious/spiritual practice that brings you closer to a Higher Power/God?

- Do you set a time aside every day to devote to your religious/spiritual practice?

- Do you find comfort in praying?

- Do you prefer to pray alone or in a group?

- Some people integrate meditation into their spiritual practices. Do you meditate?

- Do you enjoy nature?

- What is your concept of God?

- What do you think happens after one dies?

- Do you think we are "more than a body"?

- What specific people are important in your life?

- Have you had a spiritual/religious leader?

- Are you fulfilled with your life?

- Do you feel your spirituality gives you a purpose in life?

- How important is it in your life to attend a religious service?

- How do you describe suffering?

- Do you like children?

- Do you enjoy music?

- How do you express your feelings?

- Do you like to be hugged?

- Are you angry with somebody?

- Do you find spirituality to be a source of strength or hope? If not, mention what are your sources of hope and strength.

- What are your thoughts about the future?

- When do you feel most peaceful?

EMBRACING SPIRITUALITY

Explore with your clients whether they engage in any of the following spiritual practices:

- Prayer
- Spiritual reading
- Visualization
- Meditation

You can guide them into the different practices that would help them develop their spiritual dimension. Many ways to include any of these techniques are available and several will be covered briefly here.

The Power of Prayer

If your client does not believe in prayer, it is important you respect his beliefs, even if you pray. One cannot impose any belief. However, you can always explore this possibility as the power of prayer has been embrace by many scholars, from physicians to psychologists to alternative healers. Dr. Bernie S. Siegel in his book *101 Exercises for the Soul* (2005) suggests embracing this healing practice:

Incorporate prayer into your daily life. Find a method of prayer that works for you. Communicate with the divine and pray for yourself, those you love, those you don't, and to help the world become a more peaceful and love-filled place.

At times of grief and sorrow, even when we do not "pray," the need to open our hearts and connect with a higher being (or God) may become imperative. As Joan Borysenko reminds us, *"When we are absolutely miserable, prayer is no longer a dry rote repetition. It becomes a living and vibrant cry for help."* Ask your client whether she has any particular prayer that has helped her in this process, and ask her to write it down.

A prayer that is widely used for the comfort it provides, is the Serenity Prayer, by Reinhold Niebuhr:

God grant me the serenity to accept the things I cannot change; courage to change the things I can; and wisdom to know the difference. Living one day at a time; Enjoying one moment at a time; Accepting hardships as the pathway to peace; Taking, as He did, this sinful world as it is, not as I would have it; Trusting that He will make all things right if I surrender to His Will; That I may be reasonably happy in this life and supremely happy with Him Forever in the next. Amen.

Spiritual Readings

Many uplifting and spiritual books are available to accompany us in times of solitude. Your clients may find solace reading different types of readings, from Psalms, poems, or spiritual books.

I have found two books enlightening and comforting, like a companion to every day of the year:

- *Embraced by the Light. Prayers & Devotion for Daily Living* (2001). Bettey J. Eadie
- *Healing After Loss. Daily Meditations for Working Through* Grief (2002). Martha Whitmore Hickman

Before suggesting any book, it is advisable to read the book or at least have a notion what it is about. It would be great to have a copy at your office, so clients can look and see whether it resonates with them.

As we progress with the principles and evolve in the process, you will notice I will be suggesting books I have recommended to my clients. In Principle VI, *Take Care of Yourself,* I have included a list of books that can contribute to their personal growth.

Journaling after reading spiritual books can be a significant way for clients to connect with their inner self.

STRATEGY

• VISUALIZATION •

Ask clients to try visualization and think about a place that makes them feel in peace.

If they tell you they are not good imagining, ask them to take a look at your office, then with their eyes closed, to describe what it looks like. You can also ask them to close their eyes and describe what they are wearing. This way they will get in touch with their ability to imagine things, which can be translated into visualization.

Discuss with your client what did they experience during their visualization. Where they able to picture the garden in their mind? How was it? Did they connect with their spiritual guide? How did he or she look like? Do they remember their advice?

Meditation

Because meditation is a practice I have extensively incorporated in this system of transformation, I want to expand a little more on what it is, its benefits, and the different styles it offers to its practitioners.

When your clients are grieving, they may find solace in taking time to be with themselves, connect with their spiritual dimension, and take some "me-time" (Principle II).

I offer guided mediation classes at my center in Miami, Florida, *The Center for Transforming Lives*. And I have witnessed how this practice helps clients to connect with their essence and feel more relaxed. There are many ways now to do meditations, including apps, such as "Headspace," which can be downloaded to their phones. Jack Kornfield (2008) expresses how meditation can help us when dealing with grief or challenges:

Meditation trains us to be present in each moment with awareness, with a greater sense of openness of heart, and with clearer seeing. It can help us learn how to remain more open, and it can help us learn how to love with our whole hearts—and to be unafraid to express that love. Even in our difficulties, meditation can show the possibility of being a little less attached to the inevitable ups and downs in our lives, less afraid of the changes in both pleasure and pains. Meditation helps us to learn to love well, by discovering we can open ourselves to all the aspects of our minds, to whatever is difficult, as well as to whatever is easy.

We have discovered many benefits of meditation, which can be applied in all areas of our lives. This list mentions some of these benefits:

- Reduces migraines
- Combats insomnia
- Calms anxiety and reduces panic attacks
- Lowers levels of stress hormones
- Eases depression
- Regulates the pulse
- Lowers blood pressure

Source: Adapted from *Complete Guide to Pilates Yoga Meditation & Stress Relief* (2003).

There are different ways to do meditation, such as guided meditation, mindfulness (we will expand on this concept on Principle VIII, *Live the Now*), transcendental meditation (TM), and even walking meditation, to name a few. Your clients may want to explore different methods until they find one that fits with their personality.

Help your clients incorporate meditation in their daily life. Tell them they can start with 5 minutes a day, building their practice up to 30 minutes daily.

SPIRITUAL GROWTH

Kumar (2005) considers spiritual growth an expected outcome when grieving mindfully (remember from Principle II, it is being present and aware of the pain in the grief experience).

This growth, for many people, according to Kumar, may be getting closer to God or a higher being. However, it can also happen as one develops skills toward self-realization. The three spiritual tools (or skills), I would consider essential for personal spiritual growth are love, forgiveness, and gratitude.

Your clients while going through grief may lose connection with their essence, and through these practices you can help them reconnect. Maybe this would be the time to transform their own loss and reconnect with that aspect of themselves, as a result of living in a fast paced society.

Love

We are going to start with the most powerful emotion, which is LOVE.

Despite their feelings of grief, you can remind your clients that they are able to experience love, which is the most powerful emotion. The best place to start is with oneself.

When introducing LOVE to clients as a meaningful resource, first ask them for their definition and to describe how they express it.

In the guided meditation classes I facilitate, I ask individuals to open their hearts and connect with their inner selves. This is the meditation on love.

Visualization of Love

Visualization allows our mind to create what we need the most, and the beauty is that the body accepts it as a reality. For example, if I told you to close your eyes and think of a lemon, what would come to mind? What if I told you to imagine that lemon cut in half and to put that half in your mind? Your mind has the ability to vividly imagine what you tell it to do. The body responds to this image as if it was real. This is a powerful way to encourage clients to feel love in their heart.

Create a space where they feel loved. If they tell you they have never experienced love, ask them to imagine how they would love to feel. **Remind your clients that love starts with loving themselves.** This can be challenging for some people, especially if they cannot relate to what it means. You can ask them, based on their own needs: What does LOVE mean to you?

What if they feel they were never loved? They may have been left with a feeling of not being worthy. Instead of focusing on not having received love, you can shift and ask them, "Have you ever loved someone in your life? How do you feel in giving that love?"

Instead of focusing on what they didn't get, they focus on what they gave to others. It is a shift of perspective. It is to focus on their capacity to love, instead of the lack of love.

Love, besides being an emotion, is a response that we express through our actions. It can be learned and developed with practice. We can practice love by having loving thoughts. Ask your clients to think of an image that provokes in them a feeling of love and to embrace that feeling when they feel sad, anxious, or worried.

In order to change our emotions, it is important to pay attention to our thoughts and our memories of past events (more on the power of our mind in Principle IX). Instead of remembering the bad moments, discussions or regrets, ask your client to focus on the love that was shared and then allow that emotion to enter their lives.

Writing A Letter

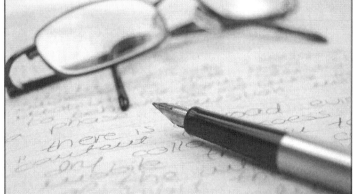

Writing letters is frequently used to express feelings through words that at times are difficult to verbalize. It is a way to connect the heart to the paper. I suggest to my clients to do it by hand on paper rather than using the computer.

These prompts or questions in the following strategy, will guide your clients in writing a letter to their loved one. Offering different entries will help them expand their own creativity and write different kinds of letters. You can also recommend they write a letter to themselves.

Clients could also decorate a box with hearts and place inside loving notes to their loved ones or to themselves. This would be beautiful activity, even for adolescents and children.

Individual or Group Activities

STRATEGY

• LETTERS TO LOVED ONES •

In writing this letter, you will be able to connect with your feelings and share them with your loved one. Keep in mind there is no right or wrong way. You may want to read these sentences, close your eyes and with all your heart, write your feelings. Do not pay attention to how you are writing; just transfer all you have in your heart to the paper.

This is releasing . . .
This is healing . . .
This is transforming. . .

Forgiveness

Forgiveness is a choice. It may not come easy for your clients, especially if they were badly hurt and keep that memory in their hearts. However, forgiveness is not about others. It is about healing oneself. Your clients may forgive someone who doesn't even know they had a grievance. Remind clients that forgiving doesn't mean forgetting, but to think about it without negativity deep in their hearts. I understand that sometimes forgiveness does not come easily because of the situation or pain that has been inflicted on us, but for clients who really want to live in peace and harmony, it is vital to be in a good spiritual place.

According to Katherine Piderman, PhD from Mayo Clinic, forgiveness can lead to:

- Healthier relationships
- Greater spiritual and psychological well-being
- Less stress and hostility
- Lower blood pressure
- Fewer symptoms of depression, anxiety, and chronic pain
- Lower risk of alcohol and substance abuse

Explore with your clients the possibility of letting go of any grudges they may have in their hearts and embracing forgiveness, love, and gratitude. Forgiveness is a powerful tool to help them develop their spiritual dimension, and sometimes your clients may have something in their heart they need to forgive, including themselves. Furthermore, it may be easier for them to forgive others than it is to forgive themselves. They may feel guilty for something they did or didn't do that could have prevented the loss they are experiencing. Forgiving oneself and others is powerful. The following exercise can help them reconcile with themselves and their humanness.

• THE POWER OF FORGIVENESS •

I wish I would have said or done . . .

_____

_____

_____

I understand I am human, therefore I forgive myself for . . .

_____

_____

_____

What do you find is the biggest challenge in forgiving that person who hurt you?

_____

_____

_____

Because I know forgiveness is a choice and I want peace in my heart I let go of . . .

_____

_____

_____

• MEDITATION •
GUIDED IMAGERY ON FORGIVENESS

I invite you to slowly take a deep breath in, and now, let it out.

Slowly take another deep breath in, and let it go.

One more time, take a deep breath in, and let it out.

So now, just take a deep breath in and inhale peace, and as you exhale, let go of any disturbing feeling you may have in your heart. Now, imagine you are carrying a backpack filled with rocks. Each rock represents a grudge or resentment. In front of you there is a steep hill. As you start climbing it, you feel how heavy the backpack is. You start letting go of the rocks from your backpack, one by one. Suddenly, even if the hill gets steeper and steeper, you feel lighter and lighter. Your backpack is so light now and you reach the top with a great sense of well-being. The same way you have let go of those rocks, you let go of any grudge or resentment you may have kept in your heart . . . you just let them go now. Stay there for a moment, breathing in and out, focusing on your breath, and when you are ready, you can slowly open your eyes.

Individual or
Group Activities

STRATEGY
• LETTER OF FORGIVENESS •

You may start a letter of forgiveness with any of these prompts:

I forgive you for . . .

I let go of my pain and forgive you for . . .

I forgive myself for . . .

I wish I would have said or done . . .

I understand I am human therefore I forgive myself for . . .

I am sorry for . . .

The hardest thing to forgive is . . .

As I forgive, I clean my soul . . .

Gratitude

> *It is this presence of thankfulness in trying times that enables us to conclude that gratitude is not a simple form of "positive thinking" or a technique of "happy-ology," but rather a deep and abiding recognition and acknowledgment that goodness exists under even the worst that life offers.*
>
> — Robert Emmons

Share with your clients this quote and ask them how they feel. They may disagree and say they do not have anything to be grateful for. In times of grief, being grateful does not come easy. When clients face the loss of a loved one or any other major life transition, gratitude may be the last resource they want to embrace. However, many studies show that being grateful helps in times of sorrow, as we learn to focus on what we have, instead of on what we have lost.

❖

Exercise

• GRATITUDE •

Reflect on the challenges to being grateful at this time in your life.

My greatest challenge is _____

_____

_____

Will I be happier if I am not grateful? _____

_____

_____

Will my life change for the better if I am not grateful? _____

_____

_____

Moving from complaint to gratitude despite losses is an opportunity to embrace the ability for spiritual growth. Do you think that is something you could feel thankful for?

Individual or Group Activities

STRATEGY

• WHAT ARE YOU THANKFUL FOR? •

Ask clients to make a list of things they are thankful for. They can start with basic needs such as having food on their plate, a roof over their heads, a bed to sleep in. Then they can move to having someone to talk to, their health, or their capacity to think. The purpose is for them to realize they have things to be grateful for.

In doing this exercise with a group, you can play some music such as *Morning Has Broken* by Cat Stevens. Despite difficult situations or losses, they can always be thankful and praise every single morning, because life is a gift.

Individual or Group Activities

STRATEGY

• A GRATITUDE JOURNAL •

Consider the following prompts:
- Thank you for . . .
- I will always be thankful for . . .
- My life is blessed because . . . I am thankful.
- What do you have to be thankful for in your life?
- Think about someone you are grateful for. How is this person? What makes you feel so grateful?
- What do you feel when you are thankful?

Encourage your clients to write down three things every night they feel grateful for. These can be simple things (e.g., they were holding a box and someone opened the door for them or someone brought them lunch). In the morning when they wake up, to read the list they wrote the night before. The following night, to write another three things they feel grateful for that day.

What will happen is that they will start paying attention to the thing to be grateful for, so they can write the list at night. This shift in perspective works. They start paying attention to the things to be grateful for. Eventually, it becomes a habit.

TRANSFORMATIVE REFLECTION

One of the main elements of developing your spirituality is the awareness that you will grow as a person, as your perception expands and you get in tune with who you really are.

The spiritual essence of human beings is a great source of strength and hope in times of crisis or loss. In this principle, I introduced three spiritual elements that may help your clients from the inside out, because the purpose is to focus on their inner resources and their ability for transformation.

It's all about opening their heart. Inviting your clients to embrace spirituality doesn't mean to be searching a strange reality, but to acquire a new quality of awareness as they discover their higher self.

EMBRACE YOUR SPIRITUALITY ACTIVITY

> *What you say to yourself counts.*
> — Dr. Bernie S. Siegel

• AFFIRMATIONS •

Now, take a deep breath, relax and close your eyes. In your mind, repeat after me, the following affirmations. Say these affirmations in a very loving and peaceful manner. You may write them down on a blank card and carry them with you.

> *I have hope for the future.*
> *Every day is an opportunity to love, to be thankful, and to forgive.*
> *I love myself and everyone else.*

This meditation is intended to be highly spiritual. If your client is religious, she can add any meaningful passage or prayer to the experience. If she does not believe in God, replace it with a word that is meaningful to her.

• MEDITATION •

Find a comfortable position and very slowly close your eyes. Take a deep breath in and let it go. Take another deep breath and let it go. One more time, take a deep breath and let it go. Now, in your mind, repeat after me:

> *In my times of distress, I just need to close my eyes and look inside myself. I seek the deepest part of my being, to charge myself with the spiritual gifts that I possess. Within me reside pure feelings that provide me with peace and hope. I let God penetrate my life and deliver me from my sorrow. I know that my faith on Him will help me move forward, step by step, along the path of my grief.*

THERAPIST EXERCISE
• SPIRITUALITY •

Do you find yourself living a spiritual life? When suggesting spiritual practices, it is always helpful to experience those practices ourselves, so we know the benefits and we can share them with our clients. If you expect your clients to process their grief and to embrace more gratitude and forgiveness in their lives, start with yourself.

How do you define spirituality? Are you spiritual?

_____

Do you practice any of the practices presented in this principle? Which one?

_____

What practice do you identify with the most? How does it help you?

_____

Do you find yourself consistent with your spiritual practices?

_____

How can these practices help you in your work with your client?

_____

Are you grateful for what you have in life?

_____

Have you forgiven people who have hurt you in the past? What about yourself?

_____

Do you love yourself?

_____

How do you feel when you teach your clients the importance of loving themselves?

_____

Chapter 7

Principle IV: Express Your Feelings

*If you keep wearing masks . . . you risk
loosing connection with yourself!*

— Ligia M. Houben

When we are happy, it is so easy to express joy. Is it easy to express grief when we are hurting inside? What about anger or guilt? Your clients may have learned to hold in their feelings. In this principle we will explore different ways to help clients express how they *really* feel.

We will show them to validate their emotions and let go of the mask they may be wearing to hide how they really feel. Once your clients are able to connect with their feelings, you can show them how to express them in an assertive way. It is important they learn how to validate those feelings instead of feeling ashamed for experiencing them.

Sometimes we assume it is easy to express our feelings. But sometimes we do not express them the way we wanted them to come out. I always ask the participants whether they are able to express their feelings. What follows are some of their comments.

DEFINITIONS OF EXPRESSING FEELINGS

For me it is difficult to say how I feel because I am scared people will tell me I am always saying I feel sad because I miss my loved one.

I was raised by a loving grandmother who told me to always love myself and to express it in taking care of my needs.

I don't have a problem saying how I feel. I took a workshop on assertiveness and learned to express my needs.

— Definitions shared in seminars or by clients

In general, our society expects a "be strong" attitude when one experiences a loss, and consequently, feelings may be repressed. At a time when so much connection is happening with the outside world, we may be risking connection with the inner self. Your clients may be risking their ability to connect with their feelings and even more, their capacity to express them.

Often, the messages we receive as children greatly influence our ability of expression. The following activity is an excellent exercise to help you understand the ability of your clients to connect with feelings and their willingness to work through them.

Meaningful Quotes

> *When you resist, repress, or deny your feelings, you disconnect yourself from your Self.*
> — Joseph Hu Dalconzo
>
> *They may forget what you said, but they will never forget how you made them feel.*
> — Carl Buechner
>
> *Focus your attention on the feelings inside you. Don't think about it, don't let your feelings turn into thinking. Stay present, and continue to be the observer of what is happening inside of you!*
> — Eckhart Tolle
>
> *Tears are the silent language of grief.*
> — Voltaire

For those clients who are disconnected with their feelings, reading a quote may be like a key to open the door to their heart. Listen with your mind and heart (as I assume you do!) and notice if there is an underlying emotion that is not being expressed.

EXERCISE

• MEANINGFUL QUOTES •

What is a meaningful quote for you? Please write it below and then answer the following questions:

_____

What does this quote mean to you?

_____

How can you apply it?

_____

What is important about this quote?

_____

Would you have changed or deleted something from the quote? What? Why?

_____

In the workshops, just before doing the activity of sharing the quotes, I like to play the song *Feelings,* by Morris Albert to create the mood of getting in touch with how they feel.

WEARING MASKS

When I do the seminars/workshops and we start Principle IV, I always say, "Raise your hand if you have ever worn a mask in your life."

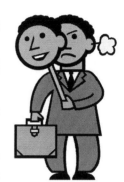

It is amazing how people relate to this experience! Everybody raises their hands!

Then, I show them an angry man, wearing the mask of a happy man.

In the workshop designed to process their personal losses, I ask people to get in pairs and I give them masks.

You can do the same, either in groups or when working with them individually. Clients tell their story of loss, first with the mask, and then without the mask. Then they process in groups how they feel. Generally, wearing a mask robs energy and can be especially draining.

If you have a mask in your office and you can do this exercise with your clients, explore how they feel and if they can relate. People need to be in touch with what they are feeling and expressing, especially with people they trust and who listen to them.

They may not be aware they are wearing masks. Many times family members and friends try to mask their pain:

Client: *It is so difficult to live without my husband . . .*

Family: *What are you saying? You look great!*

Client: *No . . . in reality, I am missing him so much.*

Family: *No! It's your idea, you are being so strong! I am so proud of you!*

Client: *You think so? That's true! You are right! I am feeling great!* (AND THEY ARE NOT)

This moment was an opportunity for clients to express how they felt. The opportunity was taken away from them. And most likely they had to wear the mask again.

People and friends want to cheer them up, they want to encourage them, telling them they are doing better when in reality they may not be doing better. Others may feel bad seeing your clients grieving.

FROM HEAD TO HEART

Your client will find it helpful if you teach them to speak from their heart, not just their head. The following strategy is how I help my clients to move from their head to their heart.

STRATEGY

• REFLECTION IN THE MIRROR •

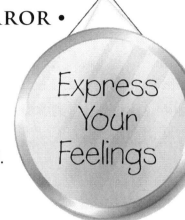

In order to share how we feel with others, it is necessary to openly express our feelings to ourselves. If your clients do not know how to openly express how they feel, you can ask them to practice in front of a mirror. In my center, I have a mirror where clients can talk to themselves and express their feelings.

Have your client say out loud in front of the mirror how they feel. They can start saying it with their eyes closed. Once they say it without hesitation, they can open their eyes and validate their feelings to themselves.

By acknowledging our feelings, we own and accept them. For your clients to be able to express their feelings freely, it is important you provide a safe place and keep a nonjudgmental stance.

Creative activities can offer a new way of releasing disturbing emotions. They can be engaging and a great way to bond with others. An activity I find to be amazing as a way to release any disturbing emotion is clapping! Yes, it is a simple activity and *easy to do*. It can also be fun, especially when you do it in a group setting.

Individual or Group Activities

STRATEGY

• RELEASING DISTURBING EMOTIONS •

Tell your client to rub their hands for a couple of minutes before starting clapping. Then, they should think about something that is disturbing for them and start clapping while focusing on that emotion.

Say the following to the group:
Take a deep breath and then let it out.
   Do this three times.
Now, start rubbing your hands.
   Do it for one minute.
NOW, start clapping.
   Clap hard, harder, harder, now (after 30 seconds) STOP!
Paying attention to your hands, separate them slowly.
Notice the flow of energy you feel BETWEEN your hands.
You can move your hands closer and separate them.
This will allow you to focus on the energy.

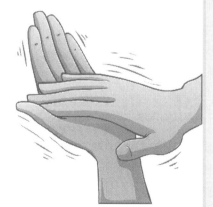

LOVING PROPS

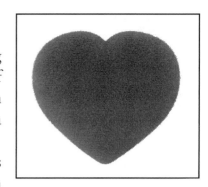

In my office I have the following objects, which I call "loving props," because they provoke in many of my clients a sense of comfort and nurture. I find them to be a great ice breaker when expressing challenging feelings. I always make sure to have a Kleenex box close to them.

When I do the workshops, I also bring them and pass them around the tables. Having the opportunity to hug them seems to be invaluable for the participants.

I remember one time when I had a bereaved mother attending the workshop. She hugged Comfee doll the entire time. She experienced a cozy feeling and was able to express her pain and tell stories about her child. It was extremely moving. We can be creative with the things we bring to workshops or have in our office.

Another object that can be useful when intense emotions, such as anger or anxiety, are experienced is a *Microbead Cushie Roll Pillow*. This pillow is great and allows clients to squeeze them and vent intense emotions without tearing them apart.

Individual or Group Activities

STRATEGY

• FELT-SENSE MEDITATION •

You may want to read this guided meditation to your client or group. Set the atmosphere by playing meditation music and lighting some candles. Ask your clients to close their eyes and relax.

Ask them to pay attention to the area between their neck and their hips and identify what they are feeling.

Where are you feeling the emotion? Is it in the heart? Is it in the stomach?

Guide them with questions than can evoke emotions as they locate them in the felt-sense area.

When are you thinking about your husband or your child?
When are you thinking about your spouse who left you?
What do you feel?

They can focus on feeling the emotion.

Then, ask them to take a deep breath in, and as they exhale to let go of that emotion.

Now take a deep breath in and as you exhale, let go of that emotion.
At this moment think about something that gives you peace. **(PAUSE)**
Now, as you have this image in your mind, repeat in your mind the word PEACE. **(PAUSE)**
Again, take a deep breath and repeat in your mind, the word PEACE. **(PAUSE)**,
One more time, take a deep breath and as you repeat in your mind the word PEACE, slowly open your eyes.

BODY SCAN

Our body and mind have a direct connection. Many times our mind is not aware of how we feel, but our body knows. Teach your clients to get in touch with how they are feeling through the messages their bodies are sending to them. One of the best ways to do it is to apply mindfulness, which will be covered extensively in Principle VIII. As we mentioned in Principle II, mindfulness is paying attention. In this case, your clients will bring mindfulness to their body. This technique is widely used in the well-known meditation method, Mindfulness-Based Stress Reduction (MBSR), created by Jon Kabat-Zinn.

The purpose is to bring awareness to the different parts of the body. Once clients focus their attention in a nonjudgmental way, ask them to notice whether any area feels uptight; then, connect with the message their body is sending to them.

STRATEGY

• FEELINGS SCAN •

As a guide to your clients, you want to help them get in touch with their emotions. Many times I ask my clients, "How do you feel?" And they respond, "I think . . ."

"No," I repeat, "how do you feel?" Then they may answer, "I believe . . ."

Ask your client to consider the following to help them move from the intellect and get in touch with their emotions:

I feel_____ when I think about my loved one.

I feel_____ when I think about my divorce.

I feel_____ when I think about getting older.

GUIDED IMAGERY

• COLOR IDENTIFICATION I •

You can add to clients' experiences by identifying a color with their emotion.

As they scan their bodies, feel the tight area, and identify the emotion, ask them:

If you were to give a color to that emotion, what would it be? Now you can dissolve the color and replace it with a color that brings peace to you.

For example, you are doing this activity with a client in private, you can ask them what is the emotion they are experiencing and the color it has. For example, if the emotion is grief and the color yellow you can say:

Now, taking a deep breath, dissolve the color yellow, and as you exhale let go of your grief.

Now ask them what color brings them peace and say the following:

Taking another deep breath and think about a color that brings peace to your soul.

They may tell you light blue or white (these are common colors people choose to feel peaceful).

Have them do breathing exercises and ask them, "What emotion would you like to feel?" For whatever emotion they name, ask them to give you a color for that emotion.

It is amazing how people begin healing with this exercise.

When you have their mind and soul in synch with imagery exercises, healing can be achieved.

EMOTIONAL COLOR

Colors, like features, follow the changes of the emotions.

— Pablo Picasso

Is there a psychology behind a color? Are we affected by colors? Research shows we tend to identify colors with moods. They have power over our feelings and how we behave. They can either give us peace or energize us. Even the colors we wear influence our mood. How can you use this resource with your clients? Besides using color in art therapy (presented in Principle II), colors can be used with different objects, including ribbons or scarves.

Guided Imagery
• Color Identification II •

Use ribbons and scarves, and code their colors.

Examples of Coding:

Red: anger   **White:** peace

Yellow: frustration   **Black:** grief

Blue: calmness   **Purple:** frustration

Green: hope

If your client is having difficulties sharing how he or she feels, ask him or her:

With what color do you identify today? Pick up a ribbon with the color that represents how you feel.

After he or she picks up the ribbon, ask him or her:

What makes you feel this way?
Now, pick up the scarf that has the color you would love to identify with and wear it.

Give him or her time to choose the scarf and put it on.

Now let me know how you feel. Get into that persona and feel the possibility of experiencing that emotion. What could you do to feel that way?

With some clients, these creative techniques may work more than just talking.

JOURNAL OF FEELINGS

Those who are grieving might think that they are grieving and sad all the time, so tell them about keeping a journal of the feelings they have throughout the day. Ask them to do it every day and at different times of the day, so if they were to wake up Monday at 7 a.m. (everyone's schedule is different), have them ask themselves, "How are you feeling this morning/afternoon/evening and/ or night?"

The most amazing thing about this practice is that they will have on paper all the emotions they felt throughout the day and week and at different times. It will also show which emotions are most relevant and help them to notice that they have other emotions. Also, it is important that once they identify the emotion, you can ask them if, for example, the emotion of peacefulness happens three times a week and what was happening at those times. Then the following week, if you see peaceful again, ask them what was happening and what they were doing that made them feel peaceful.

The important element to identify is what was happening and what were they doing at the moment of the positive emotion. We want to help them realize that the possibility of creating more positive emotions is sometimes based on what they do. One example might be when they talk to their sister and they feel understood. Maybe when they write in their journal they feel relaxed. Recognizing these correlations helps you encourage them to write more often in order to pinpoint the areas in which they were doing positive things and feeling good emotions because of it.

This practice is about creating awareness and empowering them, helping them recognize that their actions and choices help them start, little by little, to feel better and whole again. You need to get them in touch with when this is happening. Using the list of emotions, have your clients check the emotion they are feeling. They can check as many as they want. Some clients cannot express their feelings, yet when they see them on paper, they can tell you exactly the way they feel. This is another element you could add in your assessment. One of the greatest challenges the bereaved or any other type of griever may have is to find the exact word to express how they feel.

Exercise

• JOURNAL OF FEELINGS •

Keep track of feelings throughout each day. Use the list of emotions to record your feelings as precisely as you can.

	Monday	Tuesday	Wednesday	Thursday	Friday	Saturday	Sunday
7 a.m.							
10 a.m.							
1 p.m.							
4 p.m.							
7 p.m.							
10 p.m.							

LIST OF EMOTIONS

Annoyed	Depressed	Guilty	Jealous	Scared
Anxious	Embarrassed	Happy	joyful	Shy
Ashamed	Empty	Hopefull	Lonely	Sorry
Blessed	Energetic	Hopeless	Loved	Strong
Bored	Enthusiastic	Hurt	Mad	Tired
Broken	Envious	Worthless	Obessed	Upset
Cheerful	Exhaused	Worth	Proud	Worried
Confident	Frightened	Indifferent	Relieved	
Courious	Frustrated	Irritated	Sad	

PROCESSING FEELINGS

In life, we experience an array of emotions. Even if these emotions are painful, we need to validate them. There is a difference between expressing an emotion and acting on impulses motivated by emotions that may be destructive. It is believed that acting impulsively may increase the negative emotion instead of relief. An effective way to handle the emotion is doing the opposite. As we engage in the opposite behavior even our body language will change. The idea is not to deny the emotion, but to learn how to handle it or provoke a more empowering emotion (McKay, Woods, Brantley, 2007), which is why it is important to teach clients ways to deal with emotions effectively.

Emotion	Impulsive Action Based on Emotion	Opposite Behavior
Example: Anger	Hurting, insulting, withdrawing	Validating, sharing

MULTIPLE EMOTIONS

Your client may be experiencing different emotions at the same time, as they may have discovered in doing the Journal of Feelings exercise. It is normal to feel an array of emotions. What they need to do is to acknowledge and learn how to deal with them.

As uncomfortable as these emotions may feel, they are common and are experienced by many people. Although people seldom talk about them. It helps tremendously to take them out of our chest. Allow your clients to explore these feelings and to learn what has prompted them.

FACES OF EMOTIONS

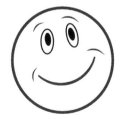 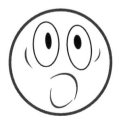   

STRATEGY

• STEM-SENTENCE •

In order to help my clients connect with their emotions at a very deep level, I use the technique Stem-Sentence as taught to me at the Institute of Interpersonal Hypnotherapy, where I studied to be a Certified Hypnotherapist. It allows the client to get in touch with how they feel regarding an event, and how the perceive themselves because of their emotions

DETERMINE EMOTIONS- "Feel so..."

Stem-Sentence Completion for Emotions:

- I isolate myself when I feel so…

- Thinking about my divorce makes me feel so…

- When I think I lost my job I feel so…

In order to get different emotions, repeat stem-sentence for 5-7 times. Notice if there are predominant emotions.

DETERMINE BELIEFS – "Like I am..."

Stem-Sentence Completion for Beliefs:

- I isolate myself when I feel so sad because I feel like I am…

- Thinking about my divorce makes me feel so angry because I feel like I am…

- When I think I lost my job I feel so frustrated because I feel like I am…

In order to get different beliefs, repeat stem-sentence for 5-7 times. Notice if there are predominant beliefs.

The final stage would be to Determine Felt-Sense.

In order to address the body felt-sense related to the emotions and beliefs, please refer to the activity on Focusing, included in Principle II.

*Adapted with permission from the Certified Hypnotherapist Program: www.InterpersonalHypnotherapy.com
This is the site for the Institute of Interpersonal Hypnotherapy founded by Matthew Brownstein, CIHt.

CHALLENGING EMOTIONS

As your clients express their grief and other emotions they may be experiencing, healing starts happening. Remind them that what they ignore doesn't cease to exist, it is only repressed.

When clients have a poor way of communicating and expressing their feelings, it is important for them to learn how to express their grief. You, as the professional, need to guide them through this process. Let them know they can communicate with others and learn to express themselves. We will elaborate on how to build communication skills in Principle V.

• AFFIRMATIONS •

The affirmations can be said every morning and every night or whenever a reminder is needed.

Now, close your eyes and in your mind, repeat after me the following affirmations. Say these affirmations in an empowered way and make them your reality. You may write them down on a blank card and carry them with you.

- *I can confront my feelings and accept them.*
- *I differentiate between anger and depression*
- *I have the ability to heal my own grief.*

• MEDITATION •

When doing this meditation, incorporate the emotions your client is experiencing and guide them to acknowledge and release any disturbing feeling they may have. Emphasize in a soothing way the words "compassionate with myself," and end it in a loving manner.

Find a comfortable position and very slowly close your eyes. Take a deep breath in and let it go. Take another deep breath and let it go. One more time, take a deep breath and let it go. Now, in your mind, repeat after me:

Living through the grieving process, I have delved into the most profound depths of my being and have embraced all my feelings, including anger, guilt, and fear. I don't need to escape from them or hide them. I understand that when I face them, I take a step closer to the transformation process. I understand that some days will be more difficult than others, but it is a process. The days that I want to cry, I will, but that does not mean that I'm going backwards on my journey of healing. I will be compassionate with myself and give myself all the time I need.

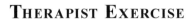

THERAPIST EXERCISE
• EXPRESSING HOW YOU FEEL •

As we work with our clients, we put all our effort in helping them express how they feel and teach them ways to feel better. What about you? Are you in touch with how you *really* feel? Do you take the time to process your emotions and notice what feelings you experience in a consistent basis or do you hide your emotions behind a mask? As you do the following exercise you will be able to express your feelings.

Are you aware of your emotions on a regular basis or do you get distracted in order not to go there?

_____

_____

Is it easier to help your client deal with their feelings than dealing with your own?

_____

_____

Which are your most prevalent emotions?

_____

_____

Describe three ways you deal with challenging emotions, such as fear, anger, or guilt.

1. _____

2. _____

3. _____

Chapter 8

Principle V: Share With Others

> *Sharing with others your loss, helps you in the healing process.*
> — Ligia M. Houben

In this principle, we continue with the transformation process. We will focus on the importance of connecting and sharing with others after facing a loss. When your clients go through grief, they may want to be by themselves and take time off. That is natural and common. However, your clients are not islands, and although they may need their "me-time," sharing with others or having "together time" could give them comfort and a space to express how they feel. We will also explore different skills and methods you can teach them to help them communicate in an effective way.

As your clients share in a meaningful way, they allow others accompany them on their path as they live through their loss.

It is about sharing. It is about connecting. It is about healing.

DEFINITIONS OF SHARING

Sharing about how one feels is an issue in my family because nobody wants to talk about it. So, being able to speak with others about how I feel, is important to me.

When I feel sad, I have a problem saying how I feel. I can only share with my loved ones, not with strangers. How could I talk in a support group?

I cannot communicate with people who interrupt when I am talking. I do not feel motivated to tell them how I feel.

Each time I share how I feel, people tell me to be strong. Then, I stay quiet. I need to find a group where I will be understood.

— Definitions shared in seminars or by clients

If you want to know how your client feels about sharing with others, you can have them express whether they find sharing easy or challenging. Keep in mind that personality plays a role in communication style, besides family dynamics. We will explore both concepts in another section of this principle. For now, the questions in the following exercise will provide a start.

❖❖
EXERCISE

• SHARING YOUR GRIEF •

How do you feel about sharing your feelings with others?

_____

_____

Does talking about your loss make you comfortable? Or does it make you feel uneasy? Why do you feel this way?

_____

_____

Is there someone in particular you feel comfortable sharing your feelings? Who is this person? How do they make you feel?

_____

_____

As you know, using quotes can be enlightening. We use them in all areas, including social media! You can show clients these quotes or ask them to look for quotes on the Internet about sharing. Ask them to bring the quotes next time they see you, or they come to group (in case you offer a support group).

Meaningful Quotes

> *Individuals with a strong social support system should be better able to cope with major life changes; those with little or no social support may be more vulnerable to life changes, particularly undesirable ones.*
>
> — Dr. Peggy A. Thoits
>
> *Pain shared is pain lessened; joy shared is joy increased.*
>
> — Spider Robinson
>
> *No wall is high or strong enough to separate us from one another's loneliness and despair. Even if we convince ourselves that we do not need other people, they need us.*
>
> — Leo F. Buscaglia

Exercise

• MEANINGFUL QUOTES •

What is a meaningful quote for you? Please write below and then answer the following questions:

_____

_____

_____

What does this quote mean to you?

_____

_____

_____

_____

How can you apply it?

_____

_____

_____

_____

What is important about this quote?

_____

_____

_____

_____

Would you have changed or deleted something from the quote? What? Why?

_____

_____

_____

_____

TEACHING YOUR CLIENT HOW TO COMMUNICATE

As a helping agent to your clients, you want to teach them skills and methods to communicate better when they are sharing with others. Their sharing will be more meaningful and effective. They will actually be heard for what they intend to say and/or they will be able to own their feelings and share them in an assertive manner.

Ask your client the following question to know how their message is coming across:

> *Have you ever experienced saying things to others they do not want to hear?*

Maybe your client has said things that are pushing people away.

For example, your client may be hurting because they feel people are not so present with their grief. They may make comments such as: *Finally you came* (or call!), or *I thought you had forgotten about me,* when someone calls or visits them.

These are comments most likely said out of pain; however, they do not induce people to continue visiting or calling. How can you teach your client to communicate better?

Remind them that people have their own lives and may be busy. So, instead of demanding their presence, what if they express how grateful they feel for their company or how much they enjoy being with them?

• HOW TO COMMUNICATE •

WHAT IF. . .

Instead of saying: *You never have time for me.*

You say: _____

Instead of saying: *I thought you had forgotten about me.*

You say: _____

Instead of saying: *Of course, you have such a busy life!*

You say: _____

Think about phrases you may have said in the past?

Instead of saying: _____

You say: _____

Instead of saying: _____

You say: _____

Respond to each of the following comments with A = always; N = never; or S = sometimes.

1. I avoid looking directly into a person's eyes.	
2. I pay attention to body language.	
3. If the person knows me well, he or she knows how I feel. I don't need to say it.	
4. Generally, I interrupt the other person to finish what he or she is saying.	
5. I ramble a lot.	
6. If I argue, I use "I" instead of "you."	
7. I talk in a direct manner. I don't allow guessing.	
8. I have a problem sharing how I feel.	
9. I don't allow anybody to know who I am.	
10. When I am with someone, I am totally present.	
11. It is a weakness to show emotions.	
12. I tend to compare my situation with others.	

Consider: If you answered **_Always_** to questions: 1, 3, 4, 5, 8, 9, 11, and 12, you may not communicate well with others. You may assume people know how you feel, do not allow them to express themselves, or you are giving different messages through verbal and body language.

FROM *YOU*-STATEMENT TO *I*-STATEMENTS

This communication tool can also be applied in groups or when working with your clients.

First, ask them to reflect on how they are expressing themselves. If they are using, I or YOU statements. Give them the following examples:

YOU-STATEMENT: You make me feel unloved when you don't pay attention to my needs.

I-STATEMENT: I feel upset when you do not take into consideration what I want or need.

Individual or Group Activities

STRATEGY

• YOU AND I STATEMENTS •

Set the group in pairs and give them a series of YOU-STATEMENTS so they can practice using I-STATEMENTS. Give each person 10 minutes. Then, ask them to choose the I-STATEMENT they want to implement in their own process.

WAYS OF COMMUNICATING

A communication style is inherent in each of us. Still, we may not be aware HOW are we communicating with the world.

In this section we will explore different ways of communicating as well as determine *your* style of communication and how you can use it to enhance the relationship and rapport with your clients. You will also teach *your client* to enhance their own communication skills. If they are grieving, the way they are communicating their grief and what they expect from others will make a difference in how they share their feeling and needs.

We all have representational systems that influences the way we communicate. In a developed country, most of us are visual (60%) and communicate with others based on our representational system. However, 20% of the population is auditory and 20% kinesthetic.

If you are leading a seminar or facilitating a group, you can ask the participants to raise their hands if they consider themselves visual. When I do this, most people raise their hands!

In NLP, we use representational systems to know how we process information and how we take what is said to us.

 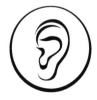 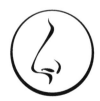 

1. Visual (V) seeing   **2.** Auditory (A) hearing   **3.** Kinesthetic (K) feeling   **4.** Olfactory (O) smelling   **5.** Gustatory (G) tasting

• REPRESENTATIONAL SYSTEMS •

Look at these words we use to express ourselves using the different representational systems, and circle the ones that apply to you.

VISUAL

Perspective
Picture
Look
Vague
Focus
Clear
Hazy
Illuminate
Scan
Vision
Bright
Lighten up
Blank
Dark
Imagine
Clarify
Colorful
Pale

AUDITORY

Quiet
Listen
Noise
Say
Talk
Tone
Harmony
Sounds
Orchestrate
Dissonance
Clicks
Resonates
Loud
Rings a bell
Whispered
Making music
Rumble
Roar

KINESTHETIC

Touch
Smooth
Grasp
Handle
Firm
Warm
Pressure
Tremble
Stir
Penetrate
Rough
Cold
Hard
Fragmented
Tapped into
Weight lifted
Solid
Blown away

OLFACTORY/ GUSTATORY

Taste
Stinks
Pungent
Scent
Odor
Whiff
Relish
Essence
Inhale
Savor
Fragrant
Sweet
Delicious
Bitter
Breath of fresh air
Sour grapes
Smell that a mile away
Spicy

Reprinted with permission. Janis Ericson, director of Lightwork Seminars Intl. Manual Neuro-Linguistic Programming (NLP), www.lightworkseminars.com.

Body Language and Actions

Your clients may not be aware they are communicating all the time, either by the words they speak, the body gestures they use, and the actions they take. If they complain to you that "nobody understands them," this activity may show them how they are processing and expressing information. It helps to practice with others how to communicate what they feel, so you can teach them more empowering ways of communicating. For example, the majority of people do not pay attention to what they convey with their gestures. If your client may be communicating something with his body that is different from his words, then showing them how easy it is to communicate without talking could make a huge difference in how his message is coming across.

I remember a client who was saying (verbally) she was happy while nodding her head and with her arms crossed. Do you think she was conveying happiness with her gestures?

If you have a group, the following activity can be done in triads. Ask the group to use different words as they communicate and to pay attention to the ones they use the most. It will indicate whether they are visual, auditory, or kinesthetic.

As the group comes together they can share what they discover about their style of communication. Is there an area they can improve for their message to come across?

GROUP STRATEGY

• COMMUNICATION STYLES •

Divide the group into triads and ask them to do the following exercise, one at a time. Each role takes 5 minutes.

#1. Shares how he/she is feeling

#2. Listens

#3. Observes the style of communication

ACTIVITY

Share with your partner something that is bothering you.

- Notice the words you use.
- Notice the gestures.
- Notice the body language.

OBSERVER

• What is the person who is sharing trying to communicate?

• How is the person doing it?

• Is that person expressing with body language the same message as the words he or she is using?

• DRAWING A WEB OF CONNECTION •

Make a list of the people you know, starting with your immediate family followed by friends, colleagues, and just acquaintances.

Once you have finished the list, plug their names in the web, and evaluate your connections.

Then share with others and, using the following questions, reflect on the connections they have in their lives.

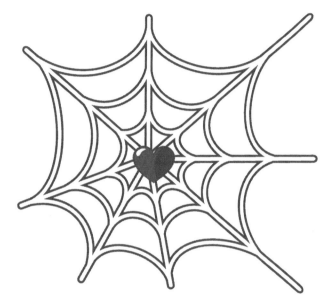

With whom do you feel more connected?

_____

What makes you feel so connected?

_____

Where you surprised by your response?

_____

How often do you share with them?

_____

In your web, decide which relationships are strong and make a commitment to engage more on a regular basis. Find ways to communicate in a better manner in the relationships you do not engage much. Is it because of you? If it's under your control, see what you can do to share more quality time with them.

WHAT DO YOU WANT TO COMMUNICATE?

At times, the bereaved expect others to know when they are needed, instead of letting people know that they need help.

People generally say to those individuals going through a loss, "Call me if you need anything." Do you think the bereaved will call? Of course not and when you ask them why not, they answer that they feel embarrassed, or do not want to be a burden to others, or that those making the offer have enough to handle.

The bereaved need help because they are grieving, especially when they have children. If someone comes offering to take their kids to school every single day, that person is giving a specific action, so the bereaved feels helped.

Now, if the question is turned around and the bereaved are asked what they expect from people (e.g., you can ask them, "What have you told others they can do?"), the clients answer that they have not told others anything, that others should know, even when that expectation maybe is not realistic. Another approach could be coming up with a strategy to describe what the bereaved needs to people who offer help. Let clients know to communicate with people and not simply expect that others will just know what is happening to your clients.

By helping them to communicate, you will help them to understand. Have your clients make a list of the things that have helped them; such a list helps them be aware of what has helped them during the grieving process or what has helped them since they encountered or suffered the loss.

Then suggest that your clients make a list of the actions and comments that have not helped. This type of awareness comes from verbalizing, and when they are talking about it, they are also healing. Maybe they have had the hurt from unhelpful commeants inside them for so long, that what you are doing for them is helping them heal by simply verbalizing it.

Also, ask your clients their preferences with others. This is important, because let's say that the bereaved does not want to do something related to the holidays and the family keeps pushing that person to do what is uncomfortable. Maybe the person wants to be in a more relaxed and calmer environment with nothing holiday related. Ask your client to describe that preference and encourage that person to share it with family and friends. As per the rights for the bereaved, they have the right to tell people their preferences, and family and friends also need to understand that this grieving is a process and what the bereaved need most is understanding, care, and love.

Individual or
Group Activities

STRATEGY

• LISTENING TO A SONG •

This activity can be done with a group (either in a support group or in a workshop).

Play the song *Lean on Me* by Bill Withers and give clients these instructions:

Sit back, relax, and listen to the music with all your heart.

If you know the words, I invite you to sing along! (I also sing!).

When you hear the clapping, you can clap too!

After the songs ends, clients may choose to respond to the following questions:

Who has ever felt the need to lean on someone?

And who has been able to lean on someone?

Judging from the responses I get, people want to share, because most of them raise their hands.

It demonstrates the need for a safe space where people can share.

ANOTHER SONG ACTIVITY

If you do not want to play the song, you can share with clients the lyrics of "Lean on Me," so they could choose a phrase and share it in group. They can elaborate on how they felt with those words.

I found this section of the song to be especially powerful:

Sometimes in our lives we all have pain
We all have sorrow
But if we are wise
We know that there's always tomorrow
Lean on me, when you're not strong
And I'll be your friend
I'll help you carry on
For it won't be long
'Til I'm gonna need
Somebody to lean on.

Many people do not have that "someone" to lean on. It may be that they do not know how to reach for people or are not aware they have built a wall around themselves, not allowing others to get in. Your clients may not be communicating well how they feel or what they expect from others, because they assume people know. Sometimes people do not know. You can teach your clients to communicate in a more effective manner as they evaluate their style of communication.

When we share with others it goes two ways. What we say and what we get back in response. Sometimes when we get a bad response from others, it may be a mirror of what we say or not say.

THE VIRTUAL WORLD

We live in a time in which the Internet is a basic component of our lives. In times of loss and grief, many people turn to their computers looking for company, comment, or a presence that they may not have present with them in other ways. Is the Internet a reliable source of support?

Yes and no. As we know, on the Internet we can find anything from insightful and helpful sites, to sites that are not monitored or are not provided by a professional. On the other hand, many forums have been created by people who have experiences personal losses and want to bring support to others. I think these are wonderful sites, as long as they provide a positive message and a safe and confidential environment.

BLOGGING

A blog is a website used to communicate as a journal. It consists of entries, or posts, where people share experiences and opinions on different subjects. Most of them allow other people to share their comments, so it becomes an online sharing community.
In many blogs about grief, people can learn about the grieving process, share their experiences, and get educated on different aspects of grief.

These are some of the most popular blogs you could share with clients:

> www.griefhealingblog.com/
> www.hellogrief.org/
> www.griefrecoverymethod.com/blog
> www.grieflink.com/blog-categories

I have my own blog where I write about grief, different life transitions, and personal growth. I like to give, when possible, the message of transformation.

ligiahouben.com/ligiasblog/

Here is an example of a blog I wrote about *Grief and the Holidays.*

In a few days starts the Holiday Season which is a time when we get together with loved ones, celebrate, and enjoy the season. If you have recently suffered the loss of a loved one, this time of the year may bring a sensation of emptiness as you miss the person who, physically, is no longer with us. What can you do about coping with loss during the Holidays? Are you supposed to ignore the Holidays altogether? Are you supposed to pretend you are not sad and show a happy face? Although you cannot change what has happened in your life you can still find new meaning during these special days.

Even though, you may not feel like celebrating, you can remember your loved one in a meaningful manner, and a beautiful way to do this is creating rituals. Rituals can help you keep their memories alive in your hearts. These rituals can be personal, with the family, or both. The advantage of creating a family ritual is that you can do it at the time you get together and want to honor your loved one.

These are examples of some rituals you can do:
- *Lighting a candle in remembrance as you gather with your family*
- *Sharing special memories*
- *Placing a chest in the living room where your family and friends can place an anecdote honoring the memory of your loved one.*

In many families, a designated person is in charge of the celebrations and when the time comes, this may be especially painful for the rest of the family. Still, you can be creative and start a new tradition. For example, Elissa, a Lebanese American, decided to celebrate Thanksgiving by cooking a stuffed lamb instead of the traditional turkey. She wanted to start their own tradition honoring her Lebanese father. In other families, they prefer to continue a family tradition like in the case of Hortensia, a Venezuelan, who cooks a special family dish every Christmas since her mother died. Her mother was known for her pernil de cerdo al horno (oven-roasted pork) and Hortensia has continued this tradition as her mother's legacy. The entire family feels closer to Hortensia's mother and their beloved country of Venezuela.

Although every celebration may bring memories of your loved one, the first celebration may be especially difficult and it is essential you prepare yourself in advance, to find meaning during these days. Because of this pain, many people may abuse alcohol or drugs during the Holidays, because they think or hope that by being numbed, they will feel better. Other people may rely on prescription drugs to deal with their grief, so they can deal with the arising emotions that may accompany grief, such as anxiety or depression. Others rely on their spirituality and participate in individual or communal rituals.

Finally, other people make the decision to go to counseling when they want a guide on how to manage grief, which is also known as grief work. What matters the most is to pay attention to your needs and validate your emotions. It is also important to acknowledge that besides experiencing the loss of a loved one, there are other losses or transitions that may interfere with our feeling joyful at this time of the year and are also crucial to validate. Among these transitions we may find:
- *Loss of a job, financial hardship*
- *Illness—mental and physical*

- *Loneliness, depression, and anxiety*
- *Having moved to a new town or place*
- *Anger and disharmony in the family*
- *Marriages breaking up*
- *Breakup with lover*
- *Loss of an animal companion*

Any situation is unique but the best you can do is to communicate your needs with others. You may also be able to transform this time of the year into an opportunity to be closer to your loved ones, and to be of service to others. For instance, you could share time or express your love for children. Or, what about sharing time with an older adult who may just need a hug and some attention? Despite our own pain, we can still be giving, loving, and appreciative. Remember that the best way to express how we feel goes beyond material gift. It has to do with giving from our heart. . . Always remember that, although the Holidays may be challenging times, it is also an opportunity to share time with special people in your life.

Remember . . . as you transform your loss, you can change your life!

WHAT ABOUT SOCIAL MEDIA?

We are living fast-paced times! Since I started working with clients and doing seminars, the world of social media has evolved tenfold! Actually, now we are all connected! Now, I ask you, as I said in one of my blogs, are we really connected? Many people are turning to the Internet to be connected with others, and they may not be connected with people close to them, or even more, with themselves! We will talk about this concept in Principle VI, which is *Take Care of Yourself* (connecting with oneself, is an essential element of taking care of oneself). However, in this section we will explore the value of social media for your clients and yourself!

If you ask around, most people engage with social media in different ways. They may have a Facebook page, a Twitter account, an Instagram page, or even a Pinterest board.

What About You?

Do you belong to any of these sites? If you do not and want to deliver your message to a broader audience, I suggest you consider joining any of these sites; social media offers a great way to share your voice. Just make sure it resonates with you and that you will be doing it consistently.

What About Your Clients and Social Media?

Many bereaved people are using the Internet in different ways: from joining support groups, to writing on blog, to sharing on Facebook or Twitter. All these ways of communicating are being used as catharsis by most, because many people are opening their heart and going public with their feelings. Moreover, they are available 24/7! How helpful is this? As stated before, the risk we are having is to disconnect with "real people." Instead of having a conversation, people may turn to their smartphones, tablets, or computers. Instead of communicating with their loved ones, they are "sharing" with strangers. However, as we explored in Chapter 3, we are unique. The way your clients process their grief is unique. Therefore, you want to know what role these elements play in the grieving process of your clients. You want to make sure they are not withdrawing from society and burying themselves in the virtual world (Social Dimension). Here comes the opportunity to have a meaningful psychoeducational moment. Remind your client of the value of connecting with others directly; a computer can never replace a human being.

PLAN ACTIVITIES

Because you want your client to connect and share with others in a meaningful way, you can suggest that they plan activities with family and friends. The following is a list of ideas.

- Have coffee together.
- Have lunch or dinner.
- Go to the movies.
- Go on vacation.
- Go to a park.
- Go to the beach.
- Watch a movie together.

- Share letters or cards.
- Go shopping for new clothes.
- Go for a massage.
- Take a cooking class.
- Take a painting class.
- Take a yoga/meditation class.
- Take a class at the university.

GROUP STRATEGY

• TELEPHONE GAME •

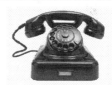

This activity is a good one, both fun and easy, to do in groups. The purpose is to show your clients/attendees how important it is not to assume people hear what we are saying. It demonstrates how easy it is to be "lost in translation" if one doesn't listen to what others are saying. We have filters that we add to what we hear. This game is an example that not everybody understands the same, so it can bring awareness to avoid judging or being resentful when people do not understand us.

- Ask the group to sit in a circle.
- The first person says something in the ear to the second person, and the second person repeats the same thing (or what she heard) to the third person.
- Members of the circle do this until the message returns to the first person. The ideal is a group with more than 6 people.
- Then, the last person in getting the message shares what she heard.

The majority of times, 9 out of 10 people hear something different from the original message!

THE VALUE OF SUPPORT GROUPS

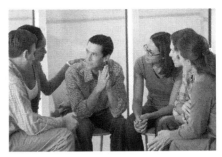

Support groups can be a safe and comforting place for your bereaved clients who are experiencing a major life transitions and need to feel accompanied in their process.

Actually, what a person needs the most when facing a loss is to be understood and heard. Support groups can offer this experience. Maybe your clients complain that their family and/or friends are telling them to "get over it ....you only talk about . . . ." They may feel alone and not validated. By belonging to a grief support group, your clients will have the opportunity to express how they feel and learn from others' stories. It will also give them the opportunity to realize they are not alone—losses happen to everybody. In addition, belonging to a support group helps to "normalize grief" when the members realize they are not going *crazy*—they are just grieving.

In communicating with others, what your clients don't want is to be told what to do. Most likely, what they want and need is to be heard. For the past 10 years, I have been training people to be facilitators of bereavement support groups in churches. I do this training with Dr. Dale Young, the director of *Congregational Health*, and the Pastoral Care department of Baptist Health South Florida, and we emphasize allowing members of the group to express how they feel, because what people need is to normalize their grief in a safe place.

Provide clients with information about support groups, even if they do not ask for it. This information is very important, especially if you work with the bereaved. They may not know there are bereavement support groups that could help them process their grief when they do not come to see you. Have a list of the groups in your area and also have information about online forums. Always make sure you check these sites to know they provide guidance and support.

Have the list handy so you can give them a copy to take with them. Remind your clients that finding a support system can be extremely valuable in their grieving process. Take a moment and look for support groups in your area. Support groups are not only for the bereaved, groups are also often available for health conditions (e.g., cancer, Alzheimer's, Parkinson's, heart conditions) and divorced people. Various groups focus on many different types of losses: job, aging, or any transition that if not handled properly can be a loss. Shifting the paradigm helps to move from grieving to embracing a new stage in life.

One of the values of support groups is that people can listen to other people's stories. It also helps to focus on others, rather than dwelling only on what has happened to them. They may think "I am the only one" before they are exposed to other people who are also facing a loss. Because they can learn a great deal from each other, sharing with others has a lot of value in the grieving and transformation process.

What about Laughing?

Is it ok to laugh in a support group?

Laughing is part of life. There is a time to cry and a time to laugh. The same way your client should not stop crying based on other's expectations ("You are crying too much!"), your client shouldn't hold in laughter based on other's expectations.

Sometimes when they start feeling happy and laughing again, clients feel guilty. It is not about the time, each one of us has our own clock. A bereavement group can also be filled with laughing— humor is a great cathartic tool. In the bereavement group, a member may share a funny story and then laugh. Because it is contagious, others laugh and may be motivated to share funny stories as well. As we know, grief is a rollercoaster, and your clients may be crying today and laughing tomorrow. Just like in life. They experience different emotions and you are there to educate them that both are part of the "normalization" of grief. The essential aspect of your guidance is to let them know they will experience an array of emotions, and that is fine. What matters most is not necessarily feeling the emotion, but what they do with it.

If you have clients who would like to attend a support group but none are available in your area, and you feel you could lead one, offer it!

Do You Offer a Support Group?

I had the privilege of contributing to the creation of the first bereavement support group, PUDE—an acronym for *Personas Unidas en el Dolor y la Esperanza* (People Joined by Pain and Hope)—in my native country of Nicaragua. This group was born after a bereaved mother, Oralí Flores, attended my seminar on how to deal with grief and loss. I had the idea of introducing the concept of bereavement support groups (an idea not embraced in Nicaragua yet), and Oralí was inspired to make it a reality. She wanted to honor her beloved daughter and at the same time help other bereaved individuals in their grieving process. I mentored her in how to put it together, and PUDE was created, using the 11 Principles of Transformation as their system to process the death of a loved one. The purpose of the group is to help people focus on their strengths, and embrace life with hope and strength.

• AFFIRMATIONS •

Affirmations can be said every morning and every night, or whenever a reminder is needed.

Now, close your eyes and in your mind, repeat after me the following affirmations. Say these affirmations in an empowered way and make them your reality. You may write them down on a blank card and carry them with you.

- *I find support in others.*
- *I realize that I am not alone.*
- *Helping others helps me in my transition.*
- *If there is someone waiting for their hand to be held, I will offer mine with love and compassion.*

This meditation is said with a tone of gratitude and appreciation. You want your client to feel grateful for having the opportunity to share with others and to feel it deep in their hearts.

• MEDITATION •

Find a comfortable position and very slowly close your eyes. Take a deep breath in and let it go. Take another deep breath and let it go. One more time, take a deep breath and let it go. Now, in your mind, repeat after me:

I am blessed because I can count on people who care about me and have offered me their hand. I have learned to share and accept the love of others. I am able to give and receive. I am able to communicate in an assertive and real way. I let others know I appreciate them and enjoy their company. I am grateful for the special people I have found on my path.

THERAPIST EXERCISE

• SHARING •

In learning about the different styles of communication you may have identified with a particular way of communicating. You may also have realized it is challenging for you to communicate what you need or want. This could be your opportunity to enhance your own communication style and then teach your clients to enhance theirs. We always teach better when we have applied our suggestions to ourselves. The following questions will help you recognize which modalities of communication presented in this chapter resonate most with you.

• Think of a time when you wished you had the support of others, what would you have liked to share?

• Do you feel comfortable sharing with others how you feel? Why or Why not?

• What is your way of communicating? Which words do you use the most?

• Are you communicating what you really feel?

Chapter 9

Principle VI: Take Care of Yourself

> *Loving yourself means taking care of your mind, body, and spirit.*
>
> — Ligia M. Houben

When your clients are facing a loss or a major life transition, they are not feeling their best emotionally and may not be paying attention to taking care of themselves. In this principle, we continue with the transformation process; however, we are moving away from focusing on grief and loss. It is not that we are ignoring the process—it is, after all, the core of the system—but now we focus more on daily living, empowerment, and the ability to look forward to brighter future.

With *Taking Care of Yourself*, your client commits to develop a positive and happier attitude for a more meaningful life. You may have clients who are so immersed in their grief that they do not feel motivated to take care of themselves. Although they may have not been able to control the loss they experienced (e.g., the death of their loved one), they can still have control over their body (a temple), their mind, which is their most powerful tool, and their spirit, which is their essence.

This principle will provide them with different suggestions on how to take care of their needs through a mind-body-spirit approach. This principle can guide your clients with specific actions they can take to connect with themselves and feel happier. They may be facing a painful loss over which they don't have control, but they can always control their actions related to their needs. Remind your clients that taking care of themselves involves paying attention to their body and mind, because a healthy body and mind take care of their spirit.

TAKING CARE OF ONESELF

It is interesting because I have always thought that taking care of myself meant I was selfish. Now I realize it is my right.

I was so impressed to learn my friend takes down time for reflection every single day, and I don't. I am inspired to take some minutes every day to reflect and see what I am doing for me. I deserve it!

When caring for others, we first need to wear the oxygen mask ourselves. It took me some time to realize I was a better caregiver for taking care of myself.

Sharing about how one feels is an issue in my family because nobody wants to talk about it. So, being able to speak with others about how I feel, is important to me.

When I feel sad, I have a problem saying how I feel. I can only share with my loved ones, not with strangers. How could I talk in a support group?

I cannot communicate with people who interrupt when I am talking. I do not feel motivated to tell them how I feel.

Each time I share how I feel, people tell me to be strong. Then, I stay quiet. I need to find a group where I will be understood.

— Definitions shared in seminars or by clients

Ask your clients to consider these questions about what taking care of themselves means.

• What does taking care of yourself mean to you?

• How would your life change if you took greater care of yourself?

Because the idea is to inspire your clients to use their inner resources to take care of themselves with strength from a deep place in their souls, you can play an uplifting song such as "Hero" by Mariah Carey and ask them to sit comfortably and relax. You can also give them a printout of the song. Here, I have included a couple of sentences your clients can use as springboard to embrace the hero they all have inside.

Hero

There's a hero
If you look inside your heart
You don't have to be afraid
Of what you are
There's an answer
If you reach into your soul
And the sorrow that you know
Will melt away
And then a hero comes along
With the strength to carry on
And you cast your fears aside
And you know you can survive

As the song says, there is a hero within each one of your clients. Sometimes they do not recognize it, but it is there. Invite clients to consider the following questions:

Do you identify with this song?

Do you feel you have a hero inside of you?

When does it come along?

How can you be your best hero?

EXERCISE

• MEANINGFUL QUOTES •

What is a meaningful quote for you? Please write it below and then answer the following questions:

_____

_____

_____

What does this quote mean to you?

_____

_____

_____

How can you apply it?

_____

_____

_____

_____

What is important about this quote?

_____

_____

_____

Would you have changed or deleted something from the quote? What? Why?

_____

_____

_____

_____

Meaningful Quotes

> *If you think taking care of yourself is selfish, change your mind.*
> *If you don't, you're simply ducking your responsibilities.*
> — Ann Richards
>
> *Emotional release and muscular release are*
> *interdependent —one does not occur without the other.*
> — Elaine Mayland
>
> *The spiritual life does not remove us from*
> *the world but leads us deeper into it.*
> — Henri J. M. Nouwen

Taking care of oneself has a different meaning to each individual. Some people find physical well-being to be their priority. Others believe their spiritual needs are the core of their lives. Some people may feel that feeding their mind with meaningful information is what brings them a sense of wellness. Although, all these perspectives are important, your clients have their own preference.

These quotes have to do with taking care at all levels: physically, mentally and spiritually. Notice which quote resonates most with them, because it will indicate their preferred dimension. You can also ask them to write a quote that inspires them to take action on the dimension they need it the most. They can write it on a small card and carry it with them all the time. Whenever they feel unmotivated to take action, they can read it for inspiration.

BODY-MIND-SPIRIT APPROACH

Inspire your client to take care of her body as it is her temple.

The Body

Before suggesting any activity or healthy lifestyle, make sure clients consult with their doctor first, so you know they are able to engage in physical activities. It may be that they complain about physical ailments due to emotional pain, however never assume it is not physical.

In this holistic approach, we start with the body. If you want to know whether your clients are taking care of their body, you can include the following worksheets in your assessment.

Your client knows what is good (and not) for them. Ask them so evaluate what they are doing with the things they can still control. Remind them, their physical care is under their control.

Even when clients share with you that they feel they cannot continue, you remind them they are taking action, because they are there with you. Remind them of their ability to take baby steps each day. To start with one, and as they evolve in their process, to add more steps. Once they start taking action and acknowledging each step, they may feel empowered and willing to continue taking more action.

WORSHEET

• DAILY ACTIVITIES •

Today's Date: _____

Hours sleeping: _____

Hours working: _____

Hours on the computer: _____

Hours eating

- Hours having breakfast: _____
- Hours having lunch: _____
- Hours having dinner: _____
- Hours having snacks: _____

Do you engage in any physical activity? _____

How many times a week?_____

By yourself or with someone? _____

How do I structure my day? _____

_____

What activities enhance my well-being? _____

_____

What activities are unhealthy?_____

_____

How does physical well-being support my inside-out transformation?

_____

What types of physical activities enhance my well-being, honor my body, and support me in this process?

_____

Take a piece of paper and write at the top, "What are my needs?" Then examine each one of them and see if you are paying attention to all of them.

WORKSHEET

• KEEP TRACK OF YOUR DAY •

Last night I went to bed at: _____ and woke up at: _____,

I woke up _____ times during the night.

How well I slept on a scale of 1–10 (1 = poorly; 10 = well rested) _____

_____

_____

_____

_____

What helps me sleep:

_____

_____

_____

_____

What keeps me awake:

_____

_____

_____

_____

What I dream about:

_____

_____

_____

_____

Exercise

Bernie S. Siegel, in his book *101 Exercises for the Soul* (2005), reminds us of a correlation between the health of our bodies and the health of our souls. Your clients can embrace this holistic approach to their well-being as they pay attention to their bodies. It can be as simple as taking a walk, which gives them the chance to get in touch with their inner selves and listen to what their heart is telling them. Keep in mind that, the most valuable message is the one your client is giving to themselves.

Benefits of Exercise

Exercise has many benefits for our physical and mental health. It can be a valuable tool in the transformation process of your clients. Once you determine where they are—whether they have a sedentary or active lifestyle—you can suggest different activities, offer resources they can use to be more active, or share with them literature that focuses on the benefits of exercise for a balanced life.

Many books, videos, and even apps for exercise are readily available. You can also review with them a list of different physical activities and ask which form of exercise resonates most. This is just an example of activities:

- Walking
- Jogging
- Pilates
- Yoga
- Spinning
- Weight lifting
- Flexibility and balance exercises
- Dance classes (e.g., Zumba)

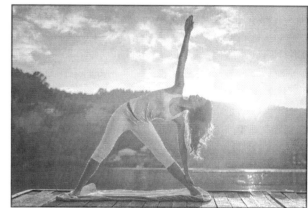

Other_____

Ask clients what types of exercises they like the most: Then encourage them to choose ONE! And to commit to start as soon as possible. You can remind them of the value of giving themselves empowering messages to motivate themselves!

Nutrition

Eating healthy and nutritious foods enhances our well-being, besides contributing to our health. Because I am not a nutritionist, I cannot recommend a specific plan to follow. Any plan should be based on the specific nutritious needs of particular clients (in case they have a health condition). However, the USDA Center on Nutrition, Policy and Promotion, provides a helpful pamphlet, "The Food Guide Pyramid," with extensive information on healthy habits.

These are their guidelines:

- Eat a variety of foods.
- Balance the food you eat with physical activity—maintain or improve your weight.
- Choose a diet with plenty of grain products, vegetables, and fruits.
- Choose a diet low in fat, saturated fat, and cholesterol.
- Choose a diet moderate in sugars.
- Choose a diet moderate in salt and sodium.
- If you drink alcoholic beverages, do so in moderation.

A great idea for your clients is to keep an eating journal or planner. They write down what they ate and how they were feeling. As we also explored earlier, grievers often eat emotionally to fill up that void created by their loss.

I found this app to be an excellent for food planning: www.foodplannerapp.com.

I suggest compile resources such as nutritionists and/or fitness instructors to provide to clients who may want or need guidelines and coaching specific to their needs.

Resting and Taking a Break

As Donald Altman states in his book, *The Mindfulness Toolbox* (2014), in times of crisis and pain, people may need to take time off and retreat into themselves. It may simply be taking a break from pain. With this in mind, I found an excellent cocoon for times when pain is just unbearable and one needs to feel protected and sheltered. It is called, the Ostrich Pillow.

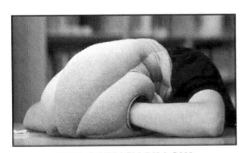

THE OSTRICH PILLOW

Pay attention to how much your client is eating, exercising, resting, and sleeping (resting can include having leisure time). You may want to review the worksheets to include in their assessments. Having balance in life has a direct effect in mood and ways of handling stress, coping with grief, and planning for the future. A tired, hungry, and cranky person cannot feel motivated and inspired for a brighter future.

Your clients may feel physically and emotionally drained by grief and loss. Their ability to think and concentrate may be impaired, as well as their energy levels. Remind them to respect their body and to take care of it—it is their temple. Self-nurture is especially important at the beginning of experiencing the loss. This includes eating well-balanced meals, resting, and finding a balance in all their activities. They need to know that caring for themselves doesn't mean feeling sorry for themselves; it means they are paying attention to their needs.

Rest-Sleep

As we saw in the dimensions of grief, insomnia can be a common expression of grief. Many people use prescription or over-the-counter drugs to help them sleep at night. Natural teas that can help them relax, such as chamomile, linden flowers, or valerian, are also available. People may use remedies such as back flowers and homeopathy. It is always advisable to check with their doctors first, in case they have any health condition or are taking medication that could have a negative effect.

Another approach to helping your clients fall asleep is by sharing with them this self-hypnosis script. You can record it and give it to them to be used at night. Remind them that they are not supposed to listen to the recording when they are driving or doing any other activity as it is extremely relaxing.

• SLEEP AND RELAXATION •
SELF-HYPNOSIS SCRIPT

Get yourself in a comfortable position lying on your bed. Take a deep breath in and as you exhale, close your eyes. Take another deep breath and exhale. Again, take a deep breath in, and say to yourself, SLEEP.

Now, you set the intention to sleep easily tonight and every night. With every single breath you take in, you become more and more sleepy. Your eyelids feel heavier and heavier, to the point that you feel you cannot open them. With your eyes closed, roll up your eyes and focus on your forehead. Imagine a soft white light on your forehead and focus on that light. You take a deep breath as you see this white and calming light, filling up your lungs with air and letting it go, thinking the word, SLEEP.

As you see this light with your inner gaze, you start counting from 5 to 1. Number 5, you see the light and feel your eyelids so heavy; number 4, you are more and more relaxed. Number 3, your eyelids are so heavy they make you feel more and more sleepy. Number 2, the weight of your eyelids feels completely comfortable. Number 1, you find yourself in the deepest feeling of relaxation, and you send this sensation of relaxation to the rest of your body, allowing this white light to fill your body from the top of your head to the tip of your toes, giving you a wave of relaxation and sleeping sensation.

As you are going deeper and deeper into your sleep, imagine you find yourself on a top of a staircase of ten steps. With every single descending step you take, you go deeper and deeper into relaxation.

Step number 10, deeper and deeper;
Step number 9, going down and down;
Step number 8, drifting into a deep sleep;
Step number 7, falling asleep so easily;
Step number 6, you are sleeping now, sleeping throughout the entire night, so easily;
Step number 5, you are sleeping so deeply, drifting deeper and deeper;
Step number 4, sleeping throughout the night; if you awake during the night, you are able to go back to sleep easily;
Step number 3, you are sleeping so well, so easily throughout the night;
Step number 2, sleeping peacefully, down and down;
Step number 1, as you go deeper and deeper, you find yourself in a beautiful garden.

In the middle of this garden you see a comfortable bed. You climb in the bed and cover yourself with a soft blanket. As you cover yourself you find a sensation of relaxation and comfort, allowing you to settle into an even deeper sleep, waking up the morning after, feeling refreshed and relaxed.

You feel your whole body relaxed, as you allow your body to fall into a deep sleep, so easily, so easily . . . sleep . . . sleep . . . going to sleep. Just by saying these words in your mind SLEEP NOW, you fall asleep so easily . . . so deeply . . . so softly . . . SLEEP NOW.

Me-Time

In times of sorrow (and also in times of joy), it is essential for your clients to have *me-time*. Do your clients think they deserve it? Do they have an idea how to do it?

It is their responsibility to take care of themselves and feel healthier and happier. In clients' *me-time* they can do whatever they like: time to reflect, exercise, do some reading, or just go for a walk.

In the following list you will find different ways clients can soothe themselves when their soul feels especially bruised. They will feel better as they pamper themselves with some "me-time."

Ask clients to choose from the following list an activity they would like to do during their me-time:

- Have a bubble bath
- Get a massage
- Do a spinning class
- Join a gym
- Cuddle up with a cup of hot tea
- Rent an old film
- Go for a walk on the beach
- Take a meditation class
- Travel to a foreign country
- Do some spring cleaning
- Get together with a group of friends
- Pray

Your client may have heard the message that paying attention to one's needs is selfish. Because it has a negative connotation, your clients may take it to an extreme, forgetting about their needs. However, when your clients give themselves some "me-time," they are not being selfish. They are simply loving themselves. Make sure you are checking in with clients to see whether they are including some me-time in their week.

Because grief can be manifested in our body, I want to bring to your attention the benefits of including somatic treatments when working with clients. Lyn Prashant, PhD, FT, CMT, an expert in the somatic aspects of grief, in her manual *The Art of Transforming Grief, Degriefing*® extensively presents the benefits of including different alternative therapies such as massage, touch therapies, and breathing.

If you believe in the power of combining different types of therapies and working with your clients in a holistic manner, you could also add to your list of contacts, information about massage therapists and body work practitioners.

ROLE IN THE FAMILY

One of the greatest determinants in how we behave is the role we have in our family. Your client may have a role as the caretaker or nurturer, so even if she is facing a loss, she may forget to take care of herself while taking care of others.

Ask clients the following questions to assess clients' attention to their needs:

- What role do you have in your family?
- Do you take care of others or do they take care of you?
- Are you able to express what you need?
- Do they honor your decisions and choices (e.g., eating healthy, joining a gym)?
- What could you start doing today to make sure you are paying attention to your needs and share these with your family in an assertive way?

I hope you take advantage of these suggestions and have your clients implement some of these ideas to increase their physical well-being. As the ancient adage states, "a sound mind in a sound body," if you want your clients to improve their sense of well-being, remind them to take care of their body.

SPIRITUAL CARE

Taking care of our spirituality is an essential element for leading a fulfilling life, and we do not need a formal religion to do so. Explore with your clients the activities they engage in to cultivate their spirit, which may include some of the following:

- Reading a book
- Meditation
- Yoga
- Writing in a journal
- Listening to music
- Going to church, temple, or a spiritual center
- Going to the beach or the countryside
- Engaging in spiritual conversation with friends

Ask your clients to do a different activity every day, and they may realize it really does not take that much effort and can bring a real difference to their souls.

Prayer

When people face a loss or transition, many turn to prayer and faith when everything else has failed. The power of faith and the power of prayer are, for many of us, the source of hope for this life and beyond. Many studies show how people use private and communal prayer to deal with difficult transitions or losses. People who prayed more were more able to develop their spirituality and to have an enhanced sense of well-being. Also, the role of faith and hope is essential to the process of finding meaning in one's life (Houben, 2009).

Meditation

This valuable spiritual tool of meditation can help us recover peace in our soul and meaning in our life. We will expand on this practice in Principle VIII: Live the Present, where we will be talking extensively about mindfulness. In the midst of pain and confusion, your clients need quiet space. Meditation is a practice that provides them with a space where they can communicate with their inner self. Different types of meditation include:

- Guided meditation
- Mindful meditation
- Breathing meditation
- Mantra meditation

It is helpful to start the meditation with progressive relaxation (expanded in Principle VIII), in which you help your clients relax every body part, starting with their feet all the way up to their heads.

Here is a meditation I found appropriate in times of grief. It is from *James Allen's Book of Meditations for Every Day in The Year*:

January Fifteenth

As the falling rain prepares the earth for the future crops of grain and fruit, so the rains of many sorrows showering upon the heart prepare and mellow it for the coming of that wisdom that perfects the mind and gladdens the heart. As the clouds darken the earth but to cool and fructify it, so the clouds of grief cast a shadow over the heart to prepare it for noble things. The hour of sorrow is the hour of reverence. It puts an end to the shallow sneer, the ribald jest, the cruel calumny; it softens the heart with sympathy, and enriches the mind with thoughtfulness. Wisdom is mainly recollection of all that was learned by sorrow.

Do not think that your sorrow will remain; it will pass away like a cloud.

Where self ends, grief passes away.

MENTAL CARE

Our minds are more powerful than we think. They drive or direct our actions. It is essential to feed your brain with positive and valuable information. Reading is a fundamental way to stimulate the mind, but take care to select stimulating and appropriate materials that can be of positive benefit. At this moment in time, it would be a good idea to read spiritual (like the one just mentioned), personal growth, and self-help books.

Here is a list of helpful books:

- *101 Exercises for the Soul* by Bernie S. Siegel
- *Think and Grow* Rich by Napoleon Hill
- *Living Life as a Thank You: The Transformative Power of Daily Gratitude* by Nina Lesowitz.
- *The Monk Who Sold His Ferrari* by Robin Sharma
- *Man's Search for Meaning* by Viktor E. Frankl
- *The 7 Habits of Highly Effective People* by Stephen Covey
- *Grieving Mindfully* by Sameet M. Kumar
- *James Allen's Book of Meditations for Every Day in the Year* by James Allen
- *Awaken the Giant Within: How to Take Immediate Control of Your Mental, Emotional, Physical and Financial Destiny!* by Anthony Robbins
- *The Road Less Traveled* by M. Scott Peck
- *As a Man Thinketh* by James Allen
- *Conversations with God* by Neale Donald Walsh
- *The Four Agreements* by Don Miguel Ruiz
- *Meditation As Medicine: Activate the Power of Your Natural Healing Force* by Dharma Singh Khalsa
- *Prescriptions for Living: Inspirational Lessons for a Joyful, Loving Life* by Bernie S. Siegel

Other activities that stimulate the mind are crosswords, puzzles, and playing cards.

• AFFIRMATIONS •

The affirmations can be said every morning and night or whenever a reminder is needed.

Now, close your eyes and in your mind, repeat after me the following affirmations. Say these affirmations in an empowered way and make them your reality. You may write them down on a blank card and carry them with you.

- *My body is my temple, and I take care of it.*
- *I nourish my body with healthy food.*
- *I embrace my spirituality.*

Meditation

As your client takes a deep breath in, you may also guide him or her to embrace a feeling of wellness and well-being. As he or she says this meditation the purpose is to bring them a sense of empowerment and control over what they are doing with their body, mind, and spirit.

• MEDITATION •

Find a comfortable position and very slowly close your eyes. Take a deep breath in and let it go. Take another deep breath and let it go. One more time, take a deep breath and let it go. Now, in your mind, repeat after me:

> *With every passing day, my body feels stronger and healthier. I feed my body with high-quality nutrition, and I exercise regularly, which makes me feel good and full of vitality. I feed my mind with meaningful information so that I can evolve as an individual. I have the power to decide the type of life I want to live. I choose a healthy life with high objectives.*

As we have explored this principle, you may have noticed the stance is one of taking action. It is an attitude of taking responsibility for their well-being. As a mental health professional, you can be a positive influence in the life of your client and suggest they take care of themselves. The purpose is to remind your client that, although they did not chose the event that happened to them, they can still choose how to take care of themselves and embrace their transformation.

• ARE YOU PAYING ATTENTION TO YOUR NEEDS? •

I know, I know. You take care of your client and you lead a busy life. Actually it is so busy that at times, you may forget to take care of yourself, don't you? It happens to many of us. However, as caregivers, we are working with others. In order to take care of others, we need to take care of ourselves. If we do not take care of ourselves, we tend to feel that our needs are not being met.

Do you take time for yourself? Do you recharge?

_____

_____

Are you sleeping and having leisure time?

_____

_____

How are your eating and exercise habits?

_____

_____

Are you doing something that brings joy to you?

_____

_____

Describe your ideal "me-time."

_____

_____

Now, reflect on how you feel, as you realize some of these needs may have been ignored.

_____

_____

Chapter 10

Principle VII: Use Rituals

> *Rituals bring significance in times of Loss.*
> *Make it special. Make it meaningful. Make it yours.*
>
> — Ligia M. Houben

A powerful tool for finding meaning during major life transition is the enactment of rituals.

A ritual is performing an action that has a special meaning to us. It helps us to interpret what happens in our lives. We are constantly engaging in secular or religious rituals, consciously or unconsciously. In the specific case of grief, rituals help to process it, heal the connection that was lost, and provide meaning for that precise event. As your clients embrace rituals, they need to make them personal and consistent.

In this principle we will explore how rituals can add a special layer to the transformation process.

DEFINITIONS OF RITUALS

A ritual for me is doing something that is special and brings meaning to my life. I prefer to do rituals by myself instead of in a group.

A ritual is something you can do, over and over again.

I never thought rituals could be secular, I always thought they were only religious. Now, I want to start exploring this action to find ways to feel closer to my deceased husband.

A ritual is separating time to do something special on a regular basis. It is a ceremony.

Something special. Something sacred. It has to be religious.

— Definitions shared in seminars or by clients

Ask your clients to define what they think a ritual is. They may be confused and have their own definition. Some may feel think it is religious and may not feel impelled to perform it. Others may think it can interfere with their own faith. Others may not be able to differentiate a ritual from a habit. You can give them the example of Thanksgiving, telling them we have dinner every day without thinking about it. That is a habit. However, we have dinner once a year that has a special meaning, which is Thanksgiving day. It is a ritual because it has a special meaning. It is important to explain your clients the difference between a habit and a ritual.

• RITUALS •

How do you define a ritual?

_____
_____
_____
_____
_____

How can you embrace rituals as a way of coping with your loss?

_____
_____
_____
_____
_____

What ideas come to you about rituals?

_____
_____
_____
_____
_____

How can you incorporate rituals in your life?

_____
_____
_____
_____
_____

Meaningful Quotes

Some chant in meditation, some practice deep, austere meditation; some worship
Him in adoration, some practice daily rituals. Some live the life of a wanderer.
— Atharva Veda

Journal writing is a voyage to the interior.
— Christina Baldwin

Fill your paper with the breathings of your heart.
— William Wordsworth

❖

EXERCISE

• MEANINGFUL QUOTES •

What is a meaningful quote for you?
Please write it below and then answer the following questions:

_____

What does this quote mean to you?

_____

How can you apply it?

_____

What is important about this quote?

_____

Would you have changed or deleted something from the quote? What? Why?

_____

CREATING RITUALS

Although clients can create their own rituals, your role as a guide is to share with them different ideas.

For example, when one lights a candle, it can be just out of habit. If one lights a candle to create a special mood, or, in the case of losing a loved one, your clients can experience it as a moment they have every night as they come to an empty house. It becomes their ritual. It is healing. It is special for them.

Rituals around Loss of A Loved One

Your clients can take a picture of their loved one and place it on a small table with a white candle. When they light the candle, they can say a prayer or intention on behalf of their loved one (e.g., for peace or release from suffering), give thanks for the love they had, and remember the eternal love they will always feel for them. When a loved one has touched our heart, that feeling stays there forever. Clients can do this ritual with different colored candles, although most people prefer white.

They can also create an altar for a loved one. Ask your clients what they would like to have on that altar. For example, if I were to create an altar to my father now, I would include his picture, candles, flowers, incense, matchbox cars (he was a car dealer and had some of these cars in his office); his keychain (I have a keychain with his motto), and his framed quotes.

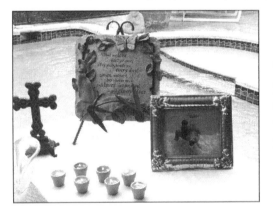

This is a beautiful example of a ritual Marlem Diaz does every year for her beloved daughter Michelle on her birthday. She always has a gathering with family and friends, and places this table in the terrace. The seven candles represent Michelle's favorite number. This action carries special meaning.

You can suggest different ideas to your clients and they can be creative, always, inspired by the love they feel in their hearts. Rituals can be individual or communal. You can ask your clients to enumerate private rituals. Many people like candles and rub lavender oil on their palms.

Rituals around Loss of Health

Candles of different colors set on a table can be assigned different kind of energies, such as vitality. Clients can rub a couple of drops of lavender oil on their temples, on the palms of their hands, and on their heart. Then, as the candles are lit, clients can imagine that their whole body is surrounded by a celestial blue light, a color that is known for its healing and spiritual powers. With faith, a call goes up for healing or to feel comfortable and in peace.

STRATEGY

• RELEASING BALLOON RITUAL •

A ritual that is used to release anger, grief, or even to connect with a deceased loved one, is to release balloons. Ask your client to get some balloons and in an open space (make sure they can release the balloons there). As the balloons get lost in the sky, clients can say out loud, "I am releasing my anger, guilt, or suffering."

You can also have a group of participants form a circle. Each participant has a balloon. As they release the balloons, they say these words, "Just like the balloons are being released, I choose now to let go of my anger. I choose peace and love in my heart."

If it is done to connect with a deceased loved one, clients can even write the name with a marker on the balloon and release it in the air. Please note, it is necessary to pick up the released balloons (to avoid environment hazard).

This ritual can also be used for divorce or any other loss that has brought emotions of anger, guilt, or fear.

STRATEGY

• BURSTING WATER BALLOONS •

I remember, as a kid, throwing water balloons in my country of Nicaragua. It was fun and playful. Now, we do it as a ritual to let go of any disturbing emotion such as anger or anxiety.

Ask participants to think about something that is provoking anger, anxiety, guilt, or fear. Then, tell them to heighten this feeling and make it really strong. Make it very intense, stronger and stronger. Tell them you will count from 1 to 3. When you say "three," they will throw the balloons making the sound, "AHHHHH!"

Rituals Around Divorce (or Breakup)

Ask clients to take a piece of paper and a pen and write a letter to their ex-husband or ex-wife. In this letter, they can let go of any feelings they may still keep in their heart, including anger or bitterness. If they need to forgive or ask for forgiveness for any action of the past they may do it as well.

Then they can tear up the letter and burn it in the candle flame. They can also tear it up and sweep it out with a broom. This can be symbolic to represent that it is out of their house and lives. This activity is meant to get rid of negative feelings that are still hurting them and preventing their progress toward recovery from their loss.

WATER AS A SYMBOL

> *They that sow in tears shall reap in joy.*
> — Psalm 126:5

An element used in many religions and spiritual ceremonies is water. For example, in Catholicism, water is used in the sacrament of Baptism, as the child is sprinkled with Holy Water. Additionally, in Hinduism, people cleanse themselves as they are immersed in the Ganges River, hoping their sins will be washed away.

In the case of grief, water can be used to cleanse the soul of the pain it feels inside, and it can be done in different ways. During a shower, many people allow their tears to come out, expressing their grief. This can be healing and can become a transformative ritual.

STRATEGY

• RITUAL OF TEARS •

Ask clients who find themselves crying while they take a shower, to close their eyes when this happens and say these words aloud:

While my tears mix with the water that is cleansing my body, my soul is being released from pain. I am able to transform my pain into joy.

STRATEGY

• SPIRITUAL BATH •

Taking a bath can also become a spiritual ritual used to release unwanted energy and achieve a sensation of lightness and renewal. Instead of taking a regular bath with soap or bathing oil, use the following ingredients:

> ¼ cup Epsom salt
> 1 tablespoon sea salt
> 12 rose petals
> ½ cup rosewater

Set the environment with candles and soft music. You could also have some lavender incense burning or lavender diffuser.

Before taking your spiritual bath, take a shower and wash yourself in a mindful way. Fill up the bathtub with warm water and add the ingredients, except the rose petals. Once you are inside of the bathtub, pour the rose petals in a mindful way. Pray for any unwanted energy to be released and allow yourself to get into a spiritual space of love and peace. Stay in the bath for 10 minutes and instead of using a towel to dry, wear a robe and allow yourself to embrace the tranquility and relaxation of this spiritual bath.

AFTER DEATH COMMUNICATION

Because the issue of communication with the deceased has emerged in several seminars, I wanted to mention a couple of rituals clients engage in to continue the bond with their loved ones in a spiritual way.

Spiritual Glass of Water

In the ritual around the loss of a loved one, some bereaved clients add a glass of water, with the belief it calls the spirits. These are Jackie's words:

> *I have a glass of water with perfume for each of my loved ones who have died. I do that to elevate their spirit. I also have a candle for Santa Bárbara and San Lázaro so they can give me strength. I have gone through a lot in life and people tell me I am a very strong woman. I suppose this has helped me.* (from *Counseling Hispanics Through Loss, Grief, and Bereavement*)

If clients share with you this belief, you can ask them, "What does this mean to you?" and allow them to elaborate. It will give them the opportunity to talk about their loss. You can use this question within all belief systems. Always remember that what matters is what they believe and what it means to them.

SIGNS

Another common way of connecting with their loved ones is to find objects, listen to a song in a special moment, or feel their presence.

The following questions will help you delve deeper with your client on this subject:

- What type of connection have you had with your loved one?
- Have you ever experienced the presence of your loved one? If so, describe that experience.
- What does this mean to you?

DREAMS

Many dream theorists (Sigmund Freud, Alfred Adler, Carl Jung, etc.) considered dreams a meaningful experience that helps us understand our lives. In dream analysis, what matters most is its interpretation. Ask clients to keep a journal on their night table, and when they wake up to record their dream and see the meaning it has in their lives.

Individual or Group Activities

STRATEGY

• BEREAVEMENT SUPPORT GROUP •

In the trainings I used to conduct with Dr. Dale Young, the former director of Pastoral Care of the Baptist Health System, we finished our time together with a ritual meant to represent past, present, and future. We gave each member a blank card and asked them to write something they want to let go of their lives. We also give them a ribbon on which they can write the name of their loved one.

While they do this, we place on a table an empty small box, a huge candle in the center, and another box filled with chocolates. These are placed in a line.

The ritual consists of placing the card of the things they want to let go in a box (representing the past, they are letting go); then, they place with a bobby pin the ribbon on the candle, representing the present, as they honor their loved one; and then, they take the chocolate of the second box, representing sweetness for their future.

Processing Grief Through Rituals

Writing a Journal

Any activity that can become a ritual: writing is processing, and as when one writes, one cleanses the soul. The process of writing is in itself a form of personal expression and, in turn, is healing, because when we write what we feel we cleanse our soul.

Your client can choose to do it in the morning as he or she wakes up or at night just before going to bed. By doing it consistently, it becomes a ritual.

Examples of entries:

- I am sad about . . .
- I fear . . .
- . . . bothers me
- I miss . . .
- I am grateful for . . .
- I hope . . .

Among the different types of journals, the one I especially like and suggest to my clients is a journal of gratitude. We covered gratitude in Principle III and we explored the positive value it can bring to the lives of our clients. The other meaningful journal is the journal of feelings we covered in Principle IV.

Writing a Letter

Letter writing has nearly become a lost art, but it provides a wonderful form of expression. Writing a letter can help the bereaved explore the following:

- Expressing love
- Forgiving
- Gratitude
- Missing you
- New beginnings
- To oneself

Scrapbooking

Scrapbooking is different from a photo album. Besides including photos, individuals can also write memories, stories, or poems to be included. They can use stickers and make designs on the pages. This ritual can be done individually or as a family. It also provides a meaningful group activity.

GROUP STRATEGY

• METAPHORICAL ACTIVITIES •

When I do the workshop to process personal losses, we do a ritual people enjoy tremendously. In it, members of the group write on a piece of paper all the times they felt guilty, angry, or fearful. After 10 minutes, a paper shredder is placed in the center of the room.

When the participants are ready, and with an empowering song (e.g., *Eye of the Tiger*, by Survivor) playing, the participants to form a line and place their list in the paper shredder.

Some do it solemnly, others dance or do it with an empowered attitude. After this activity, when asked how they feel, everybody says they feel liberated!

Even though this activity is a metaphor, it can empower them. You may have different responses based on what they are letting go. What matters the most is that they find meaning in doing this action. It is a ritual.

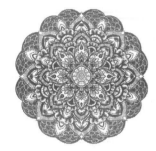

Mandalas

Susana Fisher, in her book *The Mandala Workbook: A Creative Guide for Self-Exploration, Balance, and Well-Being* (2009), explores what mandalas are, which in Sanskrit means "magic circle," and their value when facing life transitions. Mandalas offer us a profound way to examine our inner reality, to integrate that understanding with our physical selves, and to feel connected to the greater universe.

There are many ways to do mandalas. For example, Tibetan Buddhist monks create them with colored sand. People can draw them or paint them on cloth. Your clients can be inspired in different manners. The basic supplies needed for using mandalas for expression include drawing paper or construction paper, markers, colored pencils, brushes, watercolor paints, ruler, and a compass.

In Fisher's book, there's a letting go mandala, which helps to let go of emotions or things that clients may not want to continue holding in their lives or their hearts. The main point is to acknowledge what is passing. These are some of her examples:

> *Are you being asked to sacrifice something: your comfort, your dignity, your job? Whom are you letting go of? Is someone leaving, growing up, or moving away? Has a relationship come to an end? Has someone died?*

Fisher recommends burning incense or lighting a candle as an honoring ritual for what has been expressed in the mandala. Then, the mandala is put away or just burned as a releasing ritual.

There is another ritual on letting go someone shared with me in a seminar I found very powerful, as it helps to release emotions. It can be used individually or in a group setting.

Sewing a Memory Quilt

This activity can be extremely special for the bereaved to do it as a family ritual. The process can follow these steps:

- Ask your client to gather pieces of clothing of their loved one and cut them into squares.
- Have the family gather in a circle to set the intention of the ritual. Then, they start sewing.
- While they do this, they can share memories of their loved one, play favorite music, or even watch family videos.
- The purpose is to create loving quilt so they can feel the connection and honor their loved one.

This activity opens the minds and hearts of people as it brings to their awareness the rituals they already engage in and their ability to create.

Individual or Group Activities

STRATEGY

• HARD BOILED EGGS •

Ask participants to write on the shell of the egg, the name of a person or something they want to let go, and then to throw it in a garbage can, saying loudly, "I let go of_____ ."

This activity can be used, for example, with a group of divorced individuals or after losing a job.

EXERCISE

• RITUAL AWARENESS •

Share rituals that are traditional in your family.

_____

_____

_____

_____

_____

Share your favorite rituals that you observe with family and individually.

_____

_____

_____

_____

_____

CREATING RITUALS

Rituals can take many forms. Some examples of personal rituals include the following:

- Taking a bath with candles
- Writing in a journal
- Doing an action that brings back memories
- Forming a book club to meet monthly and reflect on their reading
- Monthly lunch/dinner with friends or family
- Cooking a recipe of a loved one (e.g., if your client lost her mother and she had a special recipe for the Thanksgiving turkey, using the same recipe can become a loving and meaningful ritual)
- Going to the cemetery
- Going to the beach at sunrise or sunset

Sometimes objects with special meaning can be part of a ritual. You can ask clients to choose elements from this list and then to create a ritual based on their own transition.

- Religious objects
- Toy/doll
- Books
- Candles
- Incense
- Diffuser
- Flowers

- Pillow
- Water
- Perfume
- Oil
- Letters
- Pictures
- CD or DVD

Individual or Group Activities

EXERCISE

• CREATE YOUR RITUAL •

Think about an action you can take that will give meaning to the transition you are facing now. Create a ritual that will have a special meaning to YOU. Be as creative as you want. If you want to draw the ritual, it would be wonderful.

This is my new ritual:

_____

_____

_____

My new ritual means:

_____

_____

_____

_____

RITUALS FOR TRANSITIONS

Retirement

I have a friend who attended my workshop on personal losses and knows about the value of rituals. She shared with me that now, after retirement, the simple act of washing dishes has become a ritual for her. After she washes the dishes, she places a towel on top of them to signify the end of the task. This symbolizes being able to finish a task, taking her time in a mindful and precious manner. It is meaningful for her. I thought it was beautiful and asked her if I could include it in this book. All rituals are meaningful in what they symbolize and the intention we bring to them.

Old Age

Older adults are so precious, and many times they are not honored. As presented in Chapter 2, one of the stages of development that involve many losses is old age. In the manual *Aging and Spirituality: The Fourth Dimension,* I extensively talk about the value of rituals for older adults and ways that caregivers can help them to find meaning.

> *Old age is one of the transitions during which one must learn to accept losses and new roles and to adapt to physical and mental changes. In order to find purpose in this transition, elders can engage in rituals that create personal and community meaning.* (Houben, 2009)

As one approaches old age, there are many transitions that involve letting go of independence. Relinquishing the driver's license symbolizes this transition. Among the many rituals they can do, I found letting go of their driver's license and transitioning to a nursing home to be especially meaningful. Our driver's licenses symbolize independence, autonomy, and freedom. When an elder needs to relinquish a driver's license, it represents more than being able to drive whenever they want. It represents letting go of self-reliance and a greater dependence on others. Depending on how one presents it to the older adult will determine whether this relinquishment is a bitter act or if it becomes a meaningful ritual.

If you work with adult children of aging parents, this type of ritual can be of great value. Suggest they gather as a family and bring memorabilia of the cars the elder drove, including a big poster of a favorite car. Ask the person to share stories, especially about his or her first driving experience.

A moment is taken to express gratitude for having had a car and for letting go of all the "hassles" related to driving: being stressed out in traffic, paying for gas and insurance, and efforts made for repair or maintenance. Finally, focus can be placed on the comfort of being taken to places, establishing a routine that involves different choices, and being grateful in the moment.

• AFFIRMATIONS •

The affirmations can be said every morning and every night, or whenever a reminder is needed.

Now, close your eyes and in your mind, repeat after me the following affirmations. Say these affirmations in an empowered way and make them your reality. You may write them down on a blank card and carry them with you.

- *Lighting a candle brings peace to my soul.*
- *Lighting a candle lets me feel closer to my loved one.*
- *Writing in my diary helps me cleanse my soul.*
- *Writing in my journal is a way to express what I am feeling.*
- *Prayer brings me peace and inner strength.*

• MEDITATION •

Find a comfortable position and very slowly close your eyes. Take a deep breath in and let it go. Take another deep breath and let it go. One more time, take a deep breath and let it go. Now, in your mind, repeat after me:

If I feel sad or nostalgic, I know I can find peace and serenity by creating rituals that help me find meaning and connection with my inner self. As I light a candle, I bring serenity to my life. When I write in my journal, I open my heart and pour my feelings on the paper, and this helps me in my transformation.

I allow my grief to be released and open my heart to new experiences and sensations.

THERAPIST EXERCISE

• YOUR RITUALS •

In this principle, we have elaborated in different ways your client can go deeper into their spiritual dimension. What about you? Do you find yourself living a spiritual life? When suggesting spiritual practices it is always helpful to experience those practices ourselves, so we know the benefits and we can share it with our clients. If you expect your client to process their grief, and to embrace more gratitude and forgiveness in their lives, start with yourself.

How do you define rituals?

_____

_____

Do you practice any type of personal or family ritual?

_____

_____

What is the meaning rituals have for you?

_____

_____

If you could elaborate a ritual for mental health professionals, what would it be?

_____

_____

What value would this ritual have in their lives?

_____

_____

Chapter 11

Principle VIII: Live the Present

> *Today is a gift. Be mindful as you open it.*
> — Ligia M. Houben

> *Do not dwell in the past, do not dream of the future,*
> *concentrate the mind on the present moment.*
> — The Buddha

This principle is about living in the present. It's about living in the now. It is about teaching clients to incorporate mindfulness skills in their lives.

The words of the Buddha may remind you of the technique of mindfulness; he was the person who articulated it and included it as an essential element of his teachings. For many years, I have taught World Religions at a local college in Miami, Florida. Each time I teach Buddhism, the concept of mindfulness gets a lot of attention among my students because they hear the word everywhere in our Western society.

Although there seems to be a great interest, there is also confusion about the real meaning of mindfulness. According to Dr. Daya Hewapathirane, "the real focus of Buddhism is on awakening, on coming to some insight or wisdom about our true nature. Without that, we cannot get at the real source of our suffering" (2013). I particularly like the idea of being able to transform the nature of our true self through introspection and getting in touch with the source of our essence. Mindfulness is about compassion toward ourselves and others. It is about not being distracted or sleeping, but being awake. Yes, awake to ourselves. Awake to our experiences. Awake to life.

Living in the now may be confusing to some of clients. Because we live in a fast-paced society, they may not be used to taking a pause and living in the moment. This principle is based on these premises:

• Don't dwell on the past. • Don't worry about the future. • Live in the NOW.

Please notice I am not implying that clients don't plan or think about the future. I am saying not to worry about the future, because such worry has a negative connotation. The difference between planning and worrying is significant. Worrying carries a negative connotation. Planning brings hope. It is about choices. It is about having control. In a transformation process, this practice can help clients connect with their grief and grieve mindfully, as we explored in Principle II: Live Your Grief. The difference now is the focus of attention. From grieving we move to living.

The more they are in touch with living in the moment, the easier it is for clients to let go of spending time dwelling in the past or worrying about the future.

As you show clients that living mindfully means paying attention to the now, you can also start living mindfully. Let's keep in mind that we cannot teach what we do not know. In case you do not incorporate mindfulness skills already, read this chapter with the intention of embracing it in your personal and professional life.

DEFINITIONS OF LIVING IN THE NOW

Is it possible to live in the now? I am always thinking about what happened . . .

I started taking a mindfulness meditation class and I have learned to be more in my life. I never thought it could be possible.

It is not thinking about anything else. I have tried to do it, but I always go back to the day when John left me.

— Definitions shared in seminars or by clients

Individual or Group Activities

STRATEGY

• LIVING IN THE NOW •

What is your concept of living in the now?

_____

_____

What is the nature of your true self?

_____

_____

How living in the now can help you in your grieving and transformation process?

_____

_____

Meaningful Quotes

> *Mindfulness is moment-to-moment nonjudgmental awareness, cultivated*
> *by paying attention. Mindfulness arises naturally from living.*
> — Jon Kabat-Zinn
>
> *Don't live in the past. Live now. When you are eating, eat.*
> *When you are loving, love. When you are talking with someone, talk.*
> *When you are looking at a flower, look. Catch the beauty of the moment!*
> — Leo Buscaglia
>
> *I do not want to foresee the future. I am concerned with taking care of the present.*
> *God has given me no control over the moment following.*
> — Mohandas Gandhi

EXERCISE

• MEANINGFUL QUOTES •

What is a meaningful quote for you?
Please write below and then answer the following questions:

_____

What does this quote mean to you?

_____

How can you apply it?

_____

What is important about this quote?

_____

Would you have changed or deleted something from the quote? What? Why?

_____

BEING MINDFUL, TAKING A PAUSE

Because you may have clients who have heard the word *mindfulness* but are not aware of how to apply it, it is essential you explain to them what it is and how they can use it. Use the quote from Jon Kabat-Zinn, "*Mindfulness is moment-to-moment nonjudgmental awareness, cultivated by paying attention. Mindfulness arises naturally from living,*" to explain the practice and how they can integrate it in their lives.

In order for your clients to be more present in their lives and begin embracing mindfulness, ask them to take a pause three times a day. Taking these pauses may help your clients to eventually do it without thinking. They start being present in all of their activities. Even without thinking!

Individual or Group Activities

STRATEGY

• A PAUSE FOR MINDFULNESS •

What are you experiencing now?

Take a pause and evaluate all your senses.

- What do you see?
- What do you hear?
- What do you feel in your hands?

- What do you smell?
- What do you taste?

Ask them to write down their thoughts.

> ### Individual or Group Activities
>
> #### STRATEGY
>
> ## • DON'T SPILL •
>
> You will need a glass of water almost filled to the brim and a small tray. This activity can help clients develop mindfulness as they focus on what they are doing.
>
> Ask your client to place the glass of water on the tray and to walk around the room in a concentrated manner. The purpose is to avoid water from spilling.
>
> As they focus on this task, they are mindful of their activity. This activity even prevents them from worrying or having other thoughts and focuses on doing one thing at a time, being totally present. It is living in the moment.
>
> The same way they pay attention to the glass of water, they can start paying attention to themselves, going inward, and living more consciously.

MINDFUL MEDITATION

Jon Kabat-Zinn, in his audiobook *Mindfulness for Beginners* (2006), teaches us how to develop mindfulness by eating a raisin in a mindful manner. It starts by observing the raisin, paying attention to any sound it may make, smelling and touching it, and finally putting it in your mouth. The activity is done slowly, paying full attention to each aspect.

Inspired by Kabat-Zinn, I do the following meditation when I am teaching mindfulness to clients. At the Center for Transforming Lives, I first prepare the ambiance of the room by playing soft music, dimming the lights, and displaying a picture of a beautiful sunrise on the TV.

Once everybody has arrived, I start by asking students to get comfortable on the cushion and allow themselves to relax. I give them a cotton ball with lavender oil, a ceramic heart (Principle IV on the meditation on *Love*), and a Hershey's Kiss chocolate. It is amazing how often (with newcomers) people eat the chocolate as soon as they sit down. In our society, we live so fast. They are used to living fast. I need to remind them that it will be part of their experience to slow down as a group. After ringing the bell, we begin our mindful meditation in a gentle manner.

When the exercise is finished, ask the group about their experience. Was it easy to do or challenging? What thoughts came to mind? What was the best part of the experience?

BODY SCAN TO CONNECT WITH YOUR INNER SELF

A practice that helps to increase mindfulness is body scanning meditation. Explain to your clients this will help them achieve deep relaxation and awareness of what is going on with their bodies and their emotions. In this practice they apply love and compassion to each part of their body and at the same time notice any emotion that arises as they engage in the practice. You can do it with them the first

STRATEGY

• MINDFUL MEDITATION •

In this meditation we will be involving all the senses.

Start by closing your eyes.

Take a deep breath through your nose and exhale through your mouth.
As you take another deep breath in through your nose, get in touch with the beautiful senses that God gave you.

Now, open your eyes and take a look at the screen.
Notice the colors.
Notice the shapes of the clouds: the depth of the orange sky; the different types of yellow.
See how the horizon looks.

Pay attention to what you are looking at now and to what you are seeing.
Involve the sense of your seeing.
Take your time.
Look the water at the bottom.
Look at the entire scene.
Take a good look.

Be present to what you are seeing; nothing else matters.
If any thought comes to your mind, that's ok, just pay attention to what you are seeing.
I invite you to slowly close your eyes.
Now mentally go that place in the scene; just listen (I softly touch a gong, in the midst of the soft music that is playing in the background).

Slowly open your eyes and pick up the cotton you have next to your pillow.
Bring it close to your nose and smell the lavender.
Pay attention to the sense of smell.
Lavender is known to bring relaxation and calmness.
Smell once more and then return it to where it was.

Now, pick up the heart and close your eyes.
Pay attention to the shape of the heart, the size.
Notice the rough side and the smooth side. Appreciate the heart in your hand with the sense of touch.

Return the heart to where it was and take in your hand the chocolate.
Take a look at the chocolate, notice its wrapping, color, and shape.
Now, very slowly open the Kiss, paying attention to its wrapping.
Once you have it unwrapped, bring it to your lips, and slowly put it in your mouth.
Do not chew on it.
Allow it to melt in your mouth while noticing its sweetness and the sensation it brings to you.
Just enjoy it.

This is an experience of what mindfulness is, as we involve all the senses: paying attention to what we see, smell, touch, hear, and eat. When you are ready, just open your eyes.

time, so they can practice it on a regular basis until they see you again. Suggest that they keep a journal in which they can write down about their experience: if it was easy or challenging to relax, if they have intrusive thoughts coming in that prevented them from being relaxed, or if they were so relaxed they fell asleep. The ideal is for them not to judge the experience, but embrace and utilize it as a way of developing concentration and mindfulness.

Teach your clients to get in touch with how they are feeling through the messages their body is sending to them. As we have discussed, mindfulness is paying attention. In this case, clients will bring mindfulness to their body. This technique is widely used in the well-known meditation method, Mindfulness-Based Stress Reduction (MBSR), created by Jon Kabat-Zinn. Do with them the following exercise.

> ### Individual or Group Activities
>
> #### STRATEGY
>
> # • BODY SCANNING MEDITATION •
>
> *Take a comfortable position, and pay attention to your breath.*
>
> *Notice how it comes in and out without any effort. Now, take a deep breath and as you exhale, allow your eyes to close.*
>
> *Feel the sensation of your body resting on the pillow or chair and focus your attention in your breath. Now, scan your body and determine what areas feel uptight.*
>
> *You can do this body scan from your feet to your head or from your head to your feet.*
>
> - *Do you feel tightness in any area?*
> - *What comes to mind?*
> - *What do you feel?*
> - *Go there and tell me what you feel when you experience this tightness.*
> - *What do you feel?*
> - *What emotions are you experiencing?*
> - *If you were to give a color to that emotion, what would it be?*
>
> (For example, let's say a client verbalizes a feeling of grief. Ask which color comes to mind, to which "black" might be the response. Then ask what emotion he wants to feel and the color related to that emotion, for example, peace and the color blue. Continue with the exercise.)
>
> *Take a deep breath in and inhale the positive color (blue) and exhale the negative color (black). With each breath you take in, you experience that positive emotion in your heart; each time you exhale, you feel better and better.*
>
> *Again, take a deep breath in, inhaling peace and exhaling any pain, sorrow, or grief you have had trapped in your body.*
>
> *Take a deep breath in, inhaling the positive color (blue), and now, as you exhale, exhale peace. You have now embraced the positive color as you inhale and exhale. You have been transformed.*

EMBRACING MEDITATION

If clients are not familiar with meditation, tell them to start with the following short activity.

Individual or Group Activities

STRATEGY

• EMBRACING MEDITATION •

- Choose a comfortable position and focus your attention on your breath.
- Take a breath in and out, slowly…very slowly.
- Continue doing this until you find yourself getting more and more relaxed.
- If any thought comes to your mind, you let it go like a passing cloud and focus again on your breath. If you find your mind is too busy, that's fine. Take a deep breath, and let it be.
- What you want now is to be in silence, relax your body, and focus your attention on your breath.

Mindfulness is about taking one breath at a time. Taking one breath in; letting one breath out. The easiest way to start practicing mindful meditation is to focus on the breath. If clients complain that their thoughts are intruding, remind them to focus on their breath.

As clients become more comfortable with the process, they can expand into longer meditations using the method that resonates most with them. You can briefly teach your clients each meditation. You provide guidelines so they can practice at home. The main purpose is to learn to live in the moment and create a sacred space in the midst of grief, stress, or busyness.

Types of meditation include progressive relaxation, guided meditation, and mindful meditation.

BREATHING MEDITATION

Breathing meditation is quite powerful. When clients need a special relaxation or may be feeling anxious, instruct them to sit down, relax, and do this breathing technique known as belly breathing. Ask clients how they feel. When doing this activity as a group, the room can be filled with powerful energy. As people listen to others making a strong sound, they get into the experience, exhaling each time with a louder and louder sound. This activity can be extremely releasing. After they finish the activity, clients can share how they felt. They can share the thoughts that came to their minds, and what they let go with their exhalation. This activity can be especially powerful for a support group.

Individual or
Group Activities

STRATEGY

• BREATHING MEDITATION •

Place one of your hands on your belly, keeping your eyes closed. Then, place the other hand on your chest. As you inhale, you count from 1 to 7 and at the same time you expand your belly. Feel the hand on your belly rising up and the hand on your chest remaining flat. Now, hold your breath, as you count from 1 to 4. Then, exhale, counting from 1 to 8. As your belly gets flat, you make the sound AHHHH. It is important you make the sound as your breath is releasing. Now let's do it together:

Inhale 1, 2, 3, 4, 5, 6, 7. Hold 1, 2, 3, 4. Exhale 1, 2, 3, 4, 5, 6, 7, 8. Make the sound AHHHH as you flatten your belly completely…

Again: Inhale 1, 2, 3, 4, 5, 6, 7. Hold 1, 2, 3, 4. Exhale 1, 2, 3, 4, 5, 6, 7, 8. Make the sound AHHHH as you flatten your belly completely…

One more time: Inhale 1, 2, 3, 4, 5, 6, 7. Hold 1, 2, 3, 4. Exhale 1, 2, 3, 4, 5, 6, 7, 8. Make the sound AHHHH as you flatten your belly completely…

Repeat the sequence three times and then relax.

STRATEGY

• MANTRA MEDITATION •

Follow these steps before beginning meditation:

- Choose a comfortable position.
- Find a word as a mantra (such as OM, Peace, God). Set the intention of your meditation. Be mindful when repeating the mantra in your mind.
- Practice focused concentration.
- Take in your thoughts and slowly let them go.

Ask clients whether they engage in some moments of silence. If they do not, suggest that they embrace silent moments to disconnect with the mundane world, with the outside noise, and connect with their inner self at a deep level. Suggest that they refrain from playing any music or TV. Remind them that the first step is to turn off their cell phones. This time can be me-time.

PROGRESSIVE RELAXATION

This exercise helps clients pay attention to each part of their body, just like body scanning. In this activity, as they tighten their muscles and then relax them, they also have the opportunity to release trapped emotions. It is a good practice when they feel uptight, experience insomnia, or want to practice mindfulness.

Individual or Group Activities

STRATEGY

• PROGRESSIVE RELAXATION •

Take a deep breath in and let it out.

Take a deep breath and then let it out.

As you sit on the chair, focus your attention on your feet that are resting on the floor.

Now, tighten your feet, contract them tighter and tighter, and then let that tension go.

Now, go up to your calves and shins and tighten them up; contract them tightly and then release.

Move to your thighs. Contract the muscles of your thighs tightly, and then release. Move up to your hips and buttocks as they rest on the chair and contract those muscles of your buttocks tightly, tighter, and now release.

Now move up to your torso and chest. Tighten those abdominal muscles, contracting tighter and tighter, and then release.

Focus on your arms, down to your hands and fingers. Start by making a fist, tighter and tighter so that you feel your forearms getting tight. Your whole arm, from your shoulder down to your fingers feels tighter and tighter, and now release. Then, lift your shoulder, contracting the muscle, higher and higher, and then release.

Move to the muscles of your face and tighten those muscles, becoming tighter and tighter, and then release. Let go of any tension.

Consciously let go of any tension in your body.

Remain there and relax. When you are ready, slowly close your eyes.

MINDFUL WALKING

Another type of meditation can be experienced through mindful walking. One practice can be to set yourself to take a walk once a week, totally mindful. Do not do it for aerobic benefits. Do it for soul benefits. Pay attention to your surroundings.

I suggest you watch the film *Baraka* directed by Ron Fricke. Here you will able to see a Zen monk in a mindful walking meditation in the midst of a busy city, which is presumably Tokyo, Japan.

You may want to show it to your group and have them discuss it. It is a philosophical and spiritual movie.

STRATEGY

• MINDFUL WALKING •

As you practice mindful walking, keep in mind the following suggestions:

Set your intention

Walk slower than your regular pace

Lifting and Stepping in a controlled manner

What do you notice in your body, mind, or spirit?

Are you discovering things you never saw before? Did you see neighbors? Did you stop and said hello? Did you share time with them?

Be in the moment and see how they respond.

Smile and most likely you will get a smile back (if you don't, you gave them something marvelous).

Go out to your garden and see the plants. If you hear a bird chipping, pay attention and notice how it jumps from branch to branch. Be present to the miracle of this world.

If you happen to have your journal with, you even better. Write down what you feel. Maybe follow inspiration and write a poem.

Whatever helps you be in the moment, do. You will find new things happening in your life as you open your mind and heart to the present moment.

It is the only thing we have … the NOW.

MAKING A MIND JAR

This activity is fun to do in a group. Mindfulness starts as they engage in the process of creating the jar. They can take the jar with them and practice mindfulness at home.

This activity, commonly used with children, is also quite useful with adults. It helps them become more mindful and live in the present moment.

Individual or Group Activities

STRATEGY

• MIND JAR •

The following supplies are needed for this activity.

- Clear glass jar with lid
- Water
- Glycerin
- Colored glitter (I prefer silver or gold, it looks like magic when you shake it!)
- Food coloring, optional
- Glitter glue
- Dishwashing soap

Fill the jar with hot water to a point just below the brim. Add glitter glue, food coloring, glycerin, and a couple of drops of soap. Then put the lid on tightly and shake to mix it. As you shake it, release any emotion you may have inside. Do it consciously, paying attention to the glitter in the jar. Once you stop shaking the jar, notice how the glitter settles to the bottom, just like your thoughts when you apply mindfulness in your life.

• AFFIRMATIONS •

The affirmations can be said every morning and every night, or whenever a reminder is needed.

Now, close your eyes and in your mind, repeat after me the following affirmations. Say these affirmations in an empowered way and make them your reality. You may write them down on a blank card and carry them with you.

- *I live in the now.*
- *I am present in every moment.*
- *Today I live mindfully.*

Meditation

When doing this meditation, you want to do it especially mindfully. Involve all of their senses to the experience, so you can live in the now, and in a vivid and meaningful way.

• MEDITATION •

Find a comfortable position and very slowly close your eyes. Take a deep breath in and let it go. Take another deep breath and let it go. One more time, take a deep breath and let it go. Now, in your mind, repeat after me:

Learning to live in the now helps me live fully. I have discovered that I have a source of wisdom and strength not known to me before. I appreciate every experience of every day. I listen to my inner self, letting go of any thought that may distract me. I just take a deep breath and go deeper. Living to the fullest each day makes me feel alive.

Take a deep breath in and when you are ready, open your eyes.

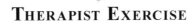

THERAPIST EXERCISE
• ARE YOU MINDFUL? •

Are you able to be present in your life? Do you pay attention to what you do in a mindful way? With this exercise, you will find out whether you are focusing on you, your life, and living moment by moment. If you are not, this is the moment to start.

Are you living in the now? Are you dwelling on past experiences or worrying about what will happen tomorrow?

_____

What does being mindful mean to you?

_____

Have you ever eaten your dinner (or lunch) without realizing when you've finished, failing to take time to savor your food?

_____

Which activity helps you be mindful? How often do you practice it?

_____

In which area of your life do you feel being mindful would add more joy and meaning?

_____

How can this practice help you in your work with your client?

_____

How can this practice help you in your life?

_____

What technique can you apply from this principle to embrace mindfulness?

_____

Chapter 12

Principle IX: Modify Your Thoughts

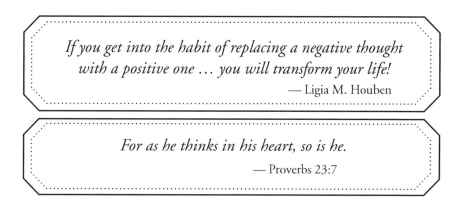

> *If you get into the habit of replacing a negative thought with a positive one ... you will transform your life!*
> — Ligia M. Houben

> *For as he thinks in his heart, so is he.*
> — Proverbs 23:7

This principle can change the lives of your clients as fast as they learn how to modify their thoughts. It is empowering. It is easy to teach. It can create breakthroughs in seconds.

Even though the idea of your clients using the power of their minds in their healing process is integrated in all principles, Principle IX focuses on how you can teach your clients to use it in concrete and empowering ways. If your clients want to change their emotions, they have to start by changing their thoughts. Notice that at this point, they have already learned to live with their grief and to express their feelings. This principle is NOT about denying feelings. It is about being aware of destructive thinking patterns and transforming them into empowering thoughts.

THE POWER OF OUR THOUGHTS

> *It is so difficult for me to stop my thoughts. Even when I try to meditate, I cannot suppress them. I wish I knew how to stop them!*
>
> *I went once to the Silva Mind Control training and they taught us to say cancel when we have a negative thought. It works when I do it, but . . . sometimes I forget it!*
>
> *I use affirmations to remind me I can think something that will help me achieve a goal.*
> — Definitions shared in seminars or by clients

Ask your client or group to share if they have times in their lives when their thoughts changed an outcome. For example, if they were facing a difficult situation, and they changed their behavior due to the message they gave to themselves, did those changes lead to a more positive outcome? They may not realize they have done this in the past, and it might be just a reminder of their ability to modify their thoughts.

❖❖

EXERCISE

• POWER OF THOUGHT •

What do you understand about the power of the mind?

_____

_____

How do you think you can you control what goes on inside your mind?

_____

_____

How do you think changing your thoughts can help you in how you see life?

_____

_____

How can you create positive changes in your life based on your thoughts?

_____

_____

Meaningful Quotes

Your life is what your thoughts make it.
— *Marcus Aurelius*

I cannot always control what goes on outside.
But I can always control what goes on inside.
— *Wayne Dyer*

You largely think the way you feel.
— *Albert Ellis*

Beliefs have the power to create and the power to destroy.
Human beings have the awesome ability to take any experience of their lives
and create a meaning that disempowers them or one that can literally save their lives.
— *Tony Robbins*

Exercise

• MEANINGFUL QUOTES •

What is a meaningful quote for you? Please write it below and then answer the following questions:

_____

_____

_____

What does this quote mean to you?

_____

_____

_____

_____

How can you apply it?

_____

_____

_____

_____

What is important about this quote?

_____

_____

_____

_____

Would you have changed or deleted something from the quote? What? Why?

_____

_____

_____

_____

MINDFUL MEDITATION ON LETTING GO OF THOUGHTS

As we have explored, mindfulness can be applied not only when meditating. Ask your clients to do the following exercise. It will allow them to be aware of the kind of thoughts they entertain in their minds. Suggest they do this in a nonjudgmental manner. They will just observe.

STRATEGY

• THOUGHT AWARENESS •

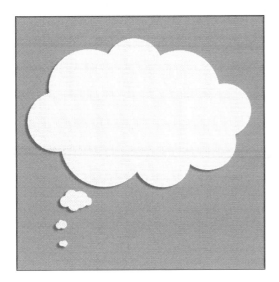

Take a deep breath and as you exhale, close your eyes. Continue breathing in and out, focusing on your breath. Be aware of your breath. Rest in the breath. Enjoy the breath.

As you focus on your breath, you may notice thoughts that come and go. That is natural. Just observe them and let them go. Take another deep breath in and let it go. When you notice another thought, just let it go as a passing cloud in a beautiful blue sky. Imagine you write the word in the cloud as it passes. Do this several times, allowing each thought to just pass by. Notice how you are able to let it go in a beautiful cloud.

When you are ready, take a deep breath in, and open your eyes.

Write down three thoughts you had during the meditation.

How did you feel when you let go of your thoughts in the cloud?

Julio Bevione (2006), in his book *Vivir en la Zona (Living in the Zone),* says that we choose how we feel, because it all originates in our mind:

Each experience you live was born out of a thought and that was your election . . . the way you feel has been your choice.

This is an essential concept for your clients to grasp. It is true they may feel sad and long for their loved one, the job they had, or how healthy they used to be. One cannot negate that reality. What they can choose is whether they want to dwell on the thought and magnify it. Based on how they think, they will feel, and based on how they feel, they will act.

If they want to start behaving in new ways, ask them to pay attention to their thoughts.

> *If you think you can do it. . .you will!*
> *Our thoughts are responsible of the result in our lives.*
> — Ligia M. Houben

In times of loss and grief, your client may have lost connection with who they are, what they are doing, or even what they are thinking. As we know, our thoughts influence how we feel; you want your clients to pause and reflect on what they are thinking and feeling.

Individual or Group Activities

STRATEGY

• ONE-MINUTE PAUSE •

If you feel a disturbing emotion, stop what you are doing and take a pause.
Pay attention in your body, where you are "feeling" the emotion, and notice what you are thinking.

Then write the thought in your journal.

At this point, what you want to do is to a greater awareness of your thoughts.
Do not judge. You are just observing.

COGNITIVE-BEHAVIORAL THERAPY

Cognitive behavioral therapy (CBT) assumes that thoughts, emotions, and behaviors are interrelated. It has proven to be an effective technique to help clients reframe their thinking so they can identify disturbing thoughts and change them into beneficial thought patterns.

> *The value of this kind of therapy is that it does not ignore the grieving process but addresses how not to perpetuate thoughts that could foster negative feelings or cause catastrophic thinking. CBT as applied to grief focuses more on helping the client move forward.*

This type of therapy has been widely implemented in a variety of challenging transitions because it provides valuable life skills and a sense of empowerment. I extensively use this technique with individuals and groups. The following is an example of how I use it with individual clients.

Across a whiteboard, I write the acronym TEA as, "THOUGHTS-EMOTIONS-ACTIONS."

When explaining what TEA means I say: **Based on what you think, you feel; and based on what you feel, you act.**

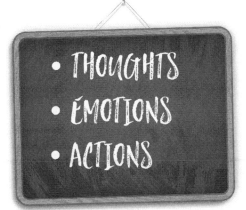

- THOUGHTS
- EMOTIONS
- ACTIONS

This explanation is followed with practicing ways to change clients' thoughts from maladaptive to empowering. The purpose is for them to realize they may have unhealthy thinking patterns that prevent them from being happier and transforming their challenges into opportunities and their losses into personal growth.

Our feelings are based on our thinking. The psychologist Shad Helmstetter is a pioneer in the power of our thoughts and the subject of self-talk. Many years ago, I read his book *What to Say When You Talk to Yourself* (1982) and have recommended it to so many clients. Dr. Helmstetter has done a great job describing ways to use positive thoughts and change old, destructive patterns of thinking. He reminds us we have control of our lives and it all starts with our inner conversation. Additionally, he wrote the book, *The Power of Neuroplasticity* (2013), where he states that with the innovation of neuroplasticity, realizing that our brain continues changing throughout our lifetime and that our thoughts play a significant role in the wiring of our brain. As we create new beliefs, we create new realities.

In applying this principle, you will teach your client the value of *reframing*—they can reframe their thoughts. Sometimes your client may engage in thinking that can be destructive and is keeping them stuck in a dark place.

Additionally, some of the messages your clients received as children from parents, society, friends, or school may be ingrained in their minds, having made those messages their beliefs. Some of these messages may influence the way they are responding to their loss and the actions they are taking in their lives.

Messages from childhood become beliefs. It doesn't mean they are correct, but they may stay with your clients. Ask them about the messages they hear, if they believe in those messages, and whether they want to change the beliefs they do not want to keep.

The most important message we can receive is the one we give to ourselves. What do you say when you talk to yourself?

• WHAT DO MESSAGES MEAN? •

Write some of the messages you have received in your life that have greatly influenced the quality of your life. Then choose which you want to keep and which you want to let go. Messages that stay in our minds become our beliefs. Remember it is your choice.

Message:
_____

Value for keeping the message:
_____
_____

Value in letting the message go:
_____
_____

Message:
_____

Value for keeping the message:
_____
_____

Value in letting the message go:
_____
_____

Message:
_____

Value for keeping the message:
_____
_____

Value in letting the message go:
_____
_____

Do clients have negative message that have been perpetuated? It is essential to remind them that they have the ability to change the messages. They have the power to reframe their thinking.

If clients want to change their emotions, they have to start changing their thoughts. Be aware that at this point, they have already lived their grief and also learned how to express their feelings. This principle is NOT about denying feelings. It is about being aware of destructive thinking patterns and transforming them into empowering thoughts.

Individual or Group Activities

Strategy

• RUBBER BAND PATTERN INTERRUPT •

Before doing this activity, ask the participants the follow: *How many of you engage in an inner conversation?*

Most likely they will laugh at the same time, they raise their hand! Then talk to them about the power of their thought over how they feel and the power they have to change those thoughts: *You allow your thoughts to get in the way and in order to break that loop we are going to use that rubber band.*

Give each participant a rubber band and use the following script:

How many of you magnify a single thought and make it powerful? How often, because of this magnified thought, does the situation become more painful or difficult?

For example, you want to let your friend know you feel hurt, and you start thinking: What for? She will not understand me. She may make fun of me. She may even stop talking to me. She may think I am so weak.

As you continue saying these things to yourself, you start feeling more and more upset.

So, something that might have initially given you some discomfort you allowed to give you anxiety, frustration, and even anger. Your thoughts took control over you.

Something that started with one simple thought was made huge through your loop thinking, making you feel overwhelmed and preventing you from talking to your friend.

Have you ever engaged in this type of thinking? This may have become your thought pattern.

However, the good news is that you can break the pattern. Start by putting the rubber band on your wrist and thinking about something that bothers you, something you have magnified in the past.

Then, the moment that the thought forms, snap the band and say, STOP!

This activity was part of my seminars about *Pattern Interrupt* when I became an NLP practitioner. This technique works really well. The purpose is for your client to interrupt the pattern of their limiting thoughts or beliefs the moment they start their pattern. Then, they give themselves the opportunity to choose how to respond. You might follow up this activity by asking, "How many of you want to be sad? Or worried, anxious, or fearful? Raise your hand." Most people will laugh, noticing that nobody raised their hands. Nobody wants to feel this way.

The difference here is not to invalidate an emotion. For example, if someone feels sad, it is natural and necessary to acknowledge the emotion. Your client could even set a certain time each day for grieving or even worrying. For example, he might set the time from 10 a.m.–11 a.m. to experience the emotion and process it. A participant in a workshop said that she "made an appointment" with her grief.

We have extensively discussed the importance of expressing feelings in Principles II and IV. Still, it is helpful for clients to embrace other emotions in their heart. One client lost her beloved mother, and she said, "I need to have a break from my grief. I cannot spend my whole day grieving." There is a difference between validating feelings of sadness and dwelling on an emotion and staying in a dark place. Therefore, what you are doing is sharing with your clients tools that can help them modify their thoughts, embrace positive emotions, and embrace life with empowerment and joy.

Individual or Group Activities

STRATEGY

• CHANGING THE IMAGE •

Ask your client to make a list of things that are pleasant. When she starts thinking a negative thought, tell her to say, "STOP!" and replace it with beautiful image, changing the thought. Have them name three to five beautiful things or images. Beautiful images can also be used as screen savers.

For example, one participant in a seminar shared that her son unexpectedly sent her pictures of her grandchildren, because he knows how much she loves them. She shared that just seeing the pictures, even if she is in a stressful situation, her emotion changes.

SELF-TALK

Pay attention to how your clients talk; their words will be a representation of their thoughts. For clients who tell you, "I cannot continue living without my loved one" their statement is based on thoughts produced by the event of that loss. Based on that thought, clients may feel hopeless, which may translate into mental/emotional paralysis or lethargic. They may not be motivated to take even baby steps in their process.

However if they can say, "I can continue living with my loved one in my heart," they may feel hopeful, empowered, and capable. Based on these feelings, they are better able to take action.

Is your client sharing with you any of the following thoughts?

- *I won't be happy again.*
- *Life is unfair.*
- *Why has this happened to me?*

These are some of the thoughts your client may entertain during moments of grief, despair, or hopelessness. It is natural to experience these emotions. Still, they can choose to dwell on their pain or bounce back after their loss. The thoughts they choose to have in their minds will make a huge difference in the outcome. I have been so touched by many of my clients who have faced painful situations and thrived despite their grief. I wanted to emphasize that people are amazingly resilient. They can choose empowering thoughts and will be able to even thrive after a loss.

Your clients need to recognize they are able to control their thoughts. This may sound challenging to them and they may respond with "I cannot do that. It is too difficult." You start there by noticing the word they used and pointing it out to them:

Did you notice the word you used? Difficult—do you think you would act differently?

What if you started saying, "I can do this!"?

I often say to my clients, "It may not be easy, but it is possible."

In helping clients, an essential component is your own belief. If you believe your clients are able to feel better, you will be able to help them. If you think (your thoughts also count) it is not possible for them to be happier, you will project those thoughts as well. Therefore, trust the ability of your clients. They may simply need someone who trusts in their ability to be happier. Be that person for them.

In order to change our present emotions it is important to pay attention to our thoughts and our memories of past events. If your clients feel sad, depressed, and only remember all the sad things that have happened in their lives, they will feel more sad or depressed. On the contrary, if they remember happy moments they can even change their brain chemistry as "the brain then takes on the same chemical patterns that were inputted at the time the happy events occurred" (Amen). Dr. Amen goes on saying this same approach can be applied when someone dies. Instead of remembering the bad moments, discussions, or regrets, focus on the love that was shared and then allow that emotion to enter your life.

If you want to change your _____,

You have to change your _____.

EXERCISE

• SWITCH OFF-ON •

We become what we think about all day long.
— Ralph Waldo Emerson

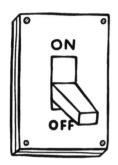

You can use a light switch to change your thoughts. Whenever you have a limiting thought, turn the switch OFF. Then, turn it ON for empowering thoughts.

Write down limiting messages – and then change them to empowering thoughts!

LIMITING

_____

_____

_____

_____

EMPOWERING

_____

_____

_____

_____

What do you think about this phrase, "When there is a will, there is a way."

_____

How can you apply it to your life now?

_____

How can you apply it to your ability to modify your thoughts?

_____

If you want to change your emotions, you have to change your thoughts.

Individual or
Group Activities

STRATEGY

• THOUGHT MODIFICATION •

Is it possible to modify your thoughts?

How do you think your life would change if you were able to change them?

CHANGING THE INNER MESSAGE

If clients are focusing on what they do not want, teach them how they can focus on what they do want. For example, if they are continually saying "I do not want to feel anxious," encourage them to change the statement to "I want to feel calm."

Your clients may also "hear" their inner talk. You can teach them to imagine a radio and use it to modify their thoughts. They will realize they can lower the volume of limiting messages and pump up the volume of empowering messages.

EXERCISE

• MOMENT OF REFLECTION •

Think of some limiting phrases you say to yourself and reframe to reflect a positive direction.

Instead of: _____

Say:_____

Instead of: _____

Say:_____

Instead of: _____

Say:_____

EXERCISE

• CHANGING OUTLOOK •

Change your mindset
Change your life
— Ligia M. Houben

Write three perspectives you have regarding your present situation and then write a new outlook, using your new inner message. Pay attention to how the words make you feel.

Your Previous Outlook	New Outlook	Difference In Your Life

JOURNAL OF THOUGHTS

Clients can keep a journal of thoughts, similar to a journal of feelings (Principle IV). They can either use that journal, the thought prior to their emotion, or TEA in this format:

- **Thought**
- **Emotion**
- **Action**

Once they record their thoughts and the effect these thoughts have on their actions, they develop awareness of how they could modify those thoughts in order to take a different type of action.

The following is an example from my book of how I introduce this concept when working with Hispanic immigrants in *Counseling Hispanics Through Loss, Grief, and Bereavement.*

Thought	Emotion	Action
I cannot adapt to this country.	Anxious	Drinking and complaining
I miss Colombia so much!	Sad	Crying
Why did I have to leave Colombia!	Angry	Snapping at spouse
English is so difficult to learn.	Afraid	Quitting school
I am so lonely here.	Sad	Being isolated

THE POWER OF METAPHORS

Metaphors are not truths in and of themselves; rather, they are pathways to truth.
— Christian Conte

A metaphor is something that symbolizes something else. Metaphor therapy is a useful technique to engage clients in learning from a story and aligning themselves with the message. A story can trigger memories or emotions that have been suppressed or ignored. As you use your skills as a caring mental health professional, you will be able to connect your clients with the message.

Let's take a famous metaphor that has been widely used. I use it with clients who choose to keep a feeling in their heart or a memory in their head. This is the story:

The Tale of Two Monks

Two monks were walking down by the river when they saw a woman waiting to cross. She was in a dress, and it was obvious she didn't want to get her dress wet. The older monk, without saying a word, picked up the woman and carried her to the other side and put her down. The two monks went on their way in complete silence. About an hour later the younger monk threw out a series of judgments to his older counterpart. "How could you have touched a woman? You know we took a vow to never touch a woman! And you didn't even seem to care to contemplate it! You just walked right over and picked her up!" The older monk listened to everything the other said and replied simply, "Brother, I put her down an hour ago, why are you still carrying her?" (Conte)

One of the most important purposes of using metaphors is to induce clients to think about the lesson or message behind the story. In this particular tale, the idea is to emphasize the value of letting go of something painful from the past. You can use this technique with individual clients or in a group.

This process begins by introducing a story: "Sit comfortably on the chair and close your eyes. Listen to the following story." At the conclusion of the story, ask listeners to take a moment to reflect and when they are ready, to share with you (or with the group) what came to mind and how they can apply it to their own story. Then, ask what it meant to them and if they need to let go in an area in their lives. I found this metaphor powerful in conveying to clients how heavy it can be to continue holding on to the past, and keeping that weight in their hearts and their minds.

In his book, *The Brain That Changes Itself: Stories of Personal Triumph from the Frontiers of Brain Science,* Norman Doidge explores the issue of grief, "Often such people cannot move on because they cannot yet grieve; the thought of living without the one they love is too painful to bear . . . we grieve by calling up one memory at a time, reliving it, and then, letting it go" (Doidge, 2007). The purpose is to guide your client into new perspectives of thinking.

> *You cannot control everything, no matter how much you try, or worry, or brood.*
> *But if you work at it, you can keep your thoughts in order. When you control*
> *your thoughts, you maintain order in your mind, body and soul.*
>
> — Bernie S. Siegel

Their thoughts will influence how they feel. The picture they have in their mind translates into how they feel and then into how they act.

The beauty is that clients can always modify their thoughts. Ask your clients whether they have an inner conversation and the tone of this conversation. Do they give to themselves empowering messages or do they have limiting beliefs? Even more, do they say to themselves things they wouldn't say to a friend? In the grieving process their thoughts play a significant role on how they transform their grief. Teach them different techniques that will empower them to make positive changes in their lives. You will be giving them the key to open the door to new opportunities, new beginnings.

I end this principle with the meaningful words of James Allen, author *As a Man Thinketh* (1902):

Mind is the Master power that moulds and makes,
And Man is Mind, and evermore he takes
The tool of Thought, and, shaping what he wills,
Brings forth a thousand joys, a thousand ills:—
He thinks in secret, and it comes to pass:
Environment is but his looking-glass.

These affirmations are to be said in an empowered and assertive way. It is helpful they write them down on a blank card and carry them around. They could even post them around the house. The purpose is for them to remind them of the power of their mind.

• AFFIRMATIONS •

Now, close your eyes and in your mind, repeat after me the following affirmations. Say these affirmations in an empowered and engaged way. They become your mantra whenever you want to feel better.

- *I make positive changes in my life.*
- *I am able to modify my thoughts.*
- *My mind is powerful.*

• MEDITATION •

Find a comfortable position and very slowly close your eyes. Take a deep breath in and let it go. Take another deep breath and let it go. One more time, take a deep breath and let it go. Now, in your mind, repeat after me:

From this moment on, I pay attention to my thoughts knowing I am able to change them. Because I want to live in harmony I embrace positive and empowering thoughts. I see my thoughts becoming a source of strength and hope. Life is beautiful and I want to live it fully. Despite pain and adversity there is a capacity in me to transform and grow. I believe in myself.

Take a deep breath in and when you are ready, open your eyes.

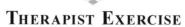

THERAPIST EXERCISE
• HOW ARE YOUR THOUGHTS? •

Are you able to change your own thoughts? In this principle we explore the way our mind influences the quality of our lives. How is your life? Do you feel empowered, positive, and hopeful? Or do you feel limited, negative, and hopeless? What are you saying to yourself?

What type of messages do you give to yourself on a regular basis?

_____

_____

Do these messages limit you or empower you?

_____

_____

Which of the strategies presented in this chapter would help you modify your thoughts?

_____

_____

How do you think your life would change if you changed your thoughts? How would you feel? What would you do differently?

_____

_____

_____

Have you done any mindful thoughts meditations?

_____

_____

What thoughts threaten to take control over you?

_____

_____

What is the most important thought you could change now to rebuild certain areas of your life?

_____

_____

Chapter 13

Principle X: Rebuild Your World

> *You are able to rebuild your world with greater meaning and purpose.*
>
> — Ligia M. Houben

The purpose in Principle X is to remind your clients they are able to rebuild their lives after a loss. This principle is about continuing to live with meaning, with their loss in their heart. When reaching this phase, they have experienced an inside-out transformation, moving through acceptance, grief, forgiveness, and hurting thoughts. They are ready now to pick up the pieces and start building the amazing gift that is their life. At this point, they may find themselves ready to continue with the process of transformation in a more meaningful way. This principle is about finding meaning in their lives and in the loss they confronted. It is a move from asking why to what for.

This principle looks at changing one's inner world despite any circumstance, just as world-renowned psychiatrist Viktor Frankl, author of *Man's Search for Meaning* did: "When we are no longer able to change a situation—we are challenged to change ourselves." We will be expanding this concept of meaning and how your clients can embrace it so they can be happier and live a meaningful life.

DEFINITIONS OF REBUILDING YOUR WORLD

I do not think I can rebuild my world without meaning. However, how can I find meaning after losing my daughter? That's why I am here.

Rebuilding my world means being able to understand what happened and continue trying. I mean, it is finding strength inside of me. Is it possible?

You say it has to do with meaning. But it is difficult to find meaning in pain. I asked myself if I wanted to become an angry person, complaining about my divorce, or if I wanted to find meaning in this new stage in my life. I decided I prefer the second option. My life changed because of this decision.

Yesterday is history. Tomorrow is a mystery. Today is a gift.

— Definitions shared in seminars or by clients

Life can be difficult at times and your clients may be facing a pain so great that they may doubt it is possible to find meaning and rebuild their world after a loss. Still, it depends on their attitude. It depends on whether they decide that despite the huge loss they have experienced, they want to transform it into personal loss. It is at this moment that the breakthrough can happen. It is at this moment when they start seeing light at the end of the tunnel, brighter and brighter. Once they find meaning and embrace life, their lives will be rebuilt little by little. What they need is a solid foundation and the desire to build a strong and meaningful life.

Trying to rebuild a world of meaning is the central process in the experience of mourning.

— Robert Neimeyer

Life consists not in holding good cards but in playing those you hold well.

— Josh Billings

Learn from yesterday, live for today, hope for tomorrow.

— Albert Einstein

You alone decide if you want to be defined by what you have lost or by who you really are.

— Dr. Bernie S. Siegel

*You are here to enable the divine purpose of the universe
to unfold. That is how important you are!*

— Eckhart Tolle

❖

EXERCISE

• MEANINGFUL QUOTES •

What is a meaningful quote for you? Please write below and then answer the following questions:

_____

What does this quote mean to you?

_____

How can you apply it?

_____

What is important about this quote?

_____

Would you have changed or deleted something from the quote? What? Why?

_____

THE VALUE OF FINDING MEANING

Meaning making is the expected outcome when working with clients. Meaning will make a difference in how they continue living. It will make a difference in how they rebuild their world after being transformed by their loss. As Robert Neimeyer, an expert in meaning-making, tells us:

Grieving is the act of affirming or reconstructing a personal world of meaning that has been challenged by loss. . . . It requires us to reconstruct a world that again "makes sense,". . . that restores a semblance of meaning, direction, and interpretability to a life that is forever transformed.

In some ways suffering ceases to be suffering at the moment it finds a meaning.

— Viktor Frankl

When we engage in existential conversation, sometimes the quality of this conversation is greatly enhanced by the sharing and bonding that can be developed within a group. Group participants can explore how this can be possible in their circumstance as they share their insights while learning about *logotherapy* and its basic tenets. This process begins by educating them about Viktor Frankl and about his seminal book, *Man's Search for Meaning.*

Viktor Frankl's Logotherapy is based on the premise that the human person is motivated by a "will to meaning," an inner pull to find a meaning in life. The following list of tenets represents basic principles of logotherapy:

- *Life has meaning under all circumstances, even the most miserable ones.*

- *Our main motivation for living is our will to find meaning in life.*

- *We have freedom to find meaning in what we do, and what we experience, or at least in the stand we take when faced with a situation of unchangeable suffering.*

REBUILDING YOUR WORLD

This principle is about helping your clients find meaning in what has happened to them as they rebuild their world with a new perspective. Its goal is to find ways to re-adjust to life and embrace it with new purpose. The world has a new order as life is reevaluated and new priorities replace old ones.

How can your clients make meaning out of what happened to them? It has to do with reframing their understanding of the situation and finding ways to transform their experience as a vehicle to contribute to the world and/or the lives of others. Once clients can make sense of their loss, their assumptive world (Chapter 2) has a new meaning. This outcome is spiritual, empowering, and meaningful. They may even discover blessings in the midst of their loss. Dr. Raymond A. Moody, in *Life After Loss: Conquering Grief and Finding Hope* (2002), indicates how there can be blessings after loss, such as *clarification of self* and *desire to serve others*, among other blessings.

Expanding on the concept of blessings, psychologists and authors Lawrence Calhoun, Jr., and Richard Tedeschi consider that posttraumatic stress can be followed by growth, which they call *strange blessings*. They presented this concept in a keynote presentation in the opening of the 2007 Association for Death Education and Counseling (ADEC) conference, with the following main types of posttraumatic growth:

- Changes in oneself—such as living a more meaningful life.
- Changes in relationships—such as forgiving someone and letting go of resentment.
- Changes in the philosophy of life—such as appreciation for every single moment and thinking that life is a gift.

You can guide clients into finding what blessings they have experienced because of their loss, focusing on the positive changes in their lives, because their loss could be the catalyst to make valuable changes in their lives.

Exercise

• Changing My Life •

What changes have you experienced after confronting this major life transition?

Yourself _____
_____
_____

Lifestyle _____
_____
_____

Relationships _____
_____
_____

Priorities _____
_____
_____

Career _____
_____
_____

Contribution to the world _____
_____
_____

Leisure _____
_____
_____

Spiritual expansion _____
_____
_____

A profound exercise clients can do is to write their own eulogy. Insight comes as they realize what is important to them, how they want to be remembered when they die, and what they are doing about it. You can also ask them to write two eulogies. To write the first eulogy as if they died today, and the second for 20 years from now. When they do this type of exercise, they can decide which choices they can make now. It is based on how they want their eulogy to be. What happens is that it may be that their ideal eulogy is not a reflection of who they are now. This is their opportunity to make those changes, the opportunity to rebuild their world with meaning and purpose.

❖

EXERCISE
• WRITING YOUR EULOGY •

My Eulogy Now

_____

_____

_____

_____

_____

_____

_____

My Eulogy in 20 Years

_____

_____

_____

_____

_____

_____

_____

_____

_____

Many Remaining Questions

Your clients may still ask questions that do not have answers. When posing these questions they may find some healing, not in knowing the why, but finding the what for.

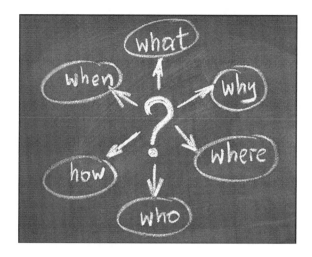

- How has my relationship to my loss evolved?
- How can I rebuild my world with this loss as part of my life, not my life?
- What am I doing now that has made the greatest impact in transforming my loss?
- Where am I standing in the journey of my life?
- How can I solidify the foundation of my life?
- What type of life do I want to build?
- Do I still have habits I need to let go in order to have a solid foundation?

GROUP STRATEGY

• USING METAPHORS IN REBUILDING •

When I conduct the workshop of the principles to transform personal losses, the group engages in different activities. The activity I do for this principle is to use LEGO blocks to rebuild clients' worlds.

As part of this activity, I play an engaging song, such as *Born to be Alive!* To begin, I place a bag of lego blocks on the top of a round table and give the following directions:

Create something. As you are able to put these blocks together, you are able to rebuild your world again.

As a team, they build a creative structure that represents how they want to rebuild their world and, above all, that they are ABLE to create the life they want, which will be presented in our last principle.

After they finish, each group can share with others what the building represents to them and how they felt during the activity. You will be surprised how creative, engaging, and dynamic this activity can be.

After this activity, invite the participants to consider which areas of their world need to be rebuilt.

The Tale of the Three Little Pigs

A tale of metaphor that works well with grieving clients is the tale of "The Three Little Pigs." The story goes that these three pigs ventured into the world on their own and wanted to build a house to protect them from the weather. They wanted a warm and safe house just like the one they had before. They decided each one of them would build a house. The first pig was thrilled and wanted to build the house *as fast as he could,* so he used the first thing that was available, which was a straw. The house was not strong, and the wolf blew it down and destroyed it. The same happened with the second pig who had built a house with wood. However, the third pig, took his time. He built it with bricks. It took longer, but he was able to create a strong house that was not blown away. It was able to withstand the wolf.

GROUP STRATEGY

• BUILDING A STRAW HOUSE •

Make copies of "The Three Little Pigs" and give it to the group. Ask one of the participants to read it and then share in group. They can brainstorm how they can build their house of bricks, using the values they have (below), and the strengths they already possess.

If some participants still want to build their house out of straw, ask them to brainstorm with the group ways to choose how to build it in bricks.

This activity works for both children and adults. The materials needed include the following:

- A box of cereal opened
- The top of a milk carton
- Glue
- Scissors
- Marker
- Brown paper
- Ashland® straw bale
(available at Michaels craft store)

Ask participants to build the walls of the house with the carton, using the top of the milk carton as the roof; then cover the carton with brown paper and straw glued to the paper. After they finish, ask them to shake the straw house and notice how feeble it is.

At this point, you could bring the LEGO blocks and have them build another house. Once they finish they can compare both and notice which feels has a stronger foundation.

Ask them, "Which foundation do you choose for your own life?"

Remember, it is all a matter of choice, and it is necessary that the choice comes from your client.

At this point, they can discard the straw house and take a picture of the LEGO building. Because this has been a group project, you can do a raffle to see which participant takes home the building. Or you could also have them do individual buildings, giving each participant a set of LEGO blocks.

Priorities In Rebuilding

As your client rebuilds his or her world after a loss or transition, that client may be reassessing priorities. Clients need to consider the following questions to gain a clear picture of what is most important for them now.

It is likely that, after facing a loss, some of your clients' values have changed and they have found new things that matter to them.

EXERCISE
• WHAT ARE YOUR PRIORITIES? •

Which of the following goals is your most important priority?

- Valuing family and friends
- Valuing myself
- Finding a purpose in my life
- Developing my spirituality
- Leaving a legacy

Where are you now in your life?

_____

_____

_____

_____

Write down three things you have learned in your process.

1._____

2._____

3._____

How have you grown as a person?

_____

_____

What have you learned?

_____

_____

See how these things have helped you become the person you are today. Use this awareness to better yourself and to build that strong foundation to continue rebuilding your world in a meaningful way.

• LIST OF VALUES •

Choose 10 values by which you either live your life or would like to live your life. From those values, choose the top three. As you rebuild your world, evaluate each area of your life and determine how you can integrate these values to provide your life with a strong and meaningful foundation.

Honesty	Loyalty	Consistency
Integrity	Nobility	Honesty
Devotion	Optimism	Authenticity
Fidelity	Grateful	Laboriousness
Equality	Happiness	Simplicity
Tolerance	Innovation	Generosity
Compassion	Maturity	Empathy
Respect	Organization	Analysis
Solidarity	Forgiveness	Gratitude
Decency	Patience	Friendship
Responsibility	Peace	Sacrifice
Justice	Personal Growth	Perseverance
Sensitivity	Professionalism	Sensibility
Discipline	Tranquility	Transparency
Sociability	Modesty	Willingness
Understanding	Dynamism	Self-Analysis
Wisdom	Sincerity	Spontaneity
Tact	Prudency	Creativity

Other value_____

LIFE REVIEW

Life may be understood backward, but it must be lived forward.

— Søren Kierkegaard

Life review is an activity in which a person takes a look into the past. Such a review is extensively used with older adults, however it can be done at any time one is facing a major life transition. As your clients engage in reminiscing, they can revise their lives and integrate their past into the present with understanding and meaning. Instead of being stuck in a painful past, they can move to find peace with forgiveness, gratitude, and love, our three spiritual tools (Principle III). At this point you want to remind your clients to integrate all the principles as they continue with their inside-out transformation.

Life reviews can be conducted in a variety of ways. In this section we will explore highs and lows and writing the chronological story.

Writing the Chronological Story

An insightful manner for conducting a life review involves asking clients to write their life story in a chronological manner. Next to each age, ask them to write a specific event that was important for them. If it was a happy memory ask them to share it with you or in the group and to experience gratitude. If it was a painful memory, help them to find ways to let it go with forgiveness, integration, and hope for the future. This activity is to be done with great love, care, and compassion from a nonjudgmental, caring, and safe place.

✦

• YOUR LIFE STORY •

Under each stage, include ages, leaving empty space to add special dates.

	Event	Emotion
Childhood		
Age:		
Age:		
Age:		
Adolescence		
Age:		
Age:		
Age:		
Adulthood		
Age:		
Age:		
Age:		
Third Age (if applicable)		
Age:		
Age:		
Age:		

EXERCISE

• HIGHS AND LOWS •

Life is a journey, filled with highs and lows, and meaning with every experience.
Chart your own history of good times and bad. See the example below to get you started.

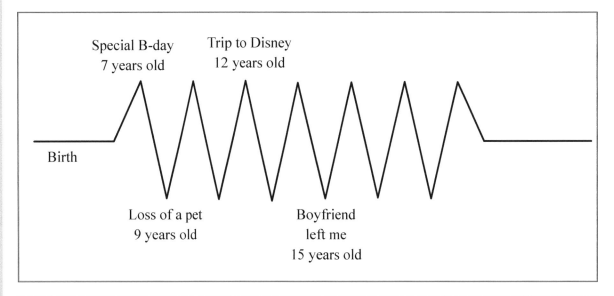

My life highs and lows

How do you feel after doing this exercise? How has recognizing happy moments helped
you to accept and transform your losses? Write a sentence that describes your awareness.

_____

_____

EXERCISE

• HISTORY OF PAST EXPERIENCE •

In the following circles, name the losses (name the ones you wrote in your "History of Losses") and wins you have had in your life. Identify the emotions linked to each experience. Notice how the mosaic of your life is painted with different colors.

Color codes: Red = Happiness   •   Black = Grief   •   Yellow = Fear   •   Green = Hope

White = Peace   •   Blue = Anxiety   •   Orange = Powerful

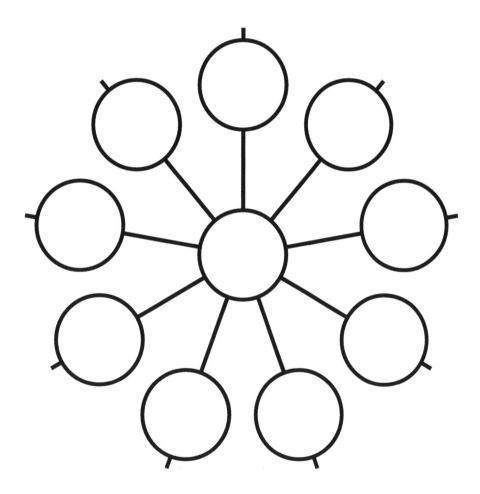

FINDING MEANING AFTER THE LOSS OF A LOVED ONE

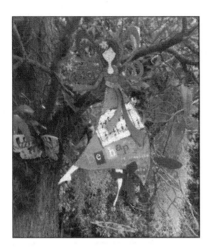

In the case of death of a loved one, one way to find meaning is to keep the memory of our loved one alive. Your clients can find different ways to do this. They can start a foundation, organization, or program. For example, if the death was caused by an accident due to a drunk driver, they might create an organization that works to prevent drunk driving.

They can also plant a tree as a symbol of continuance of life. It is a beautiful act of remembrance.

Here, I share a story of my dear client, Marlem Díaz, who has been an inspiration in how she has transformed the loss of her beloved daughter Michelle. In her story, we see the value of rituals (Principle VII) when commemorating a loved one.

A month after Michelle's passing, we planted the oak tree. Every year we gather around it to remember her, specifically on her birthday and on the anniversary of her becoming an angel. Usually on that day, December 16, since it is close to Christmas, her friends bring an ornament and we decorate the tree. We always have a toast to her beautiful life on earth around the tree.

One year, I gave her friends a white stone to write her a message and we placed them under the tree.

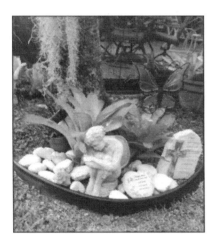

I have turned all the areas facing the tree into little corners of memories with angels, hearts, butterflies, and decorative garden stones. The tree is always seasonally decorated, since she loved to decorate for all holidays. I often sit close to it, hoping that she is there in spirit. There are a few wind chimes hanging on the tree, and every time I'm around the tree (whether or not there is wind) I hear one chime. To me it has become a place of peace and a place to connect with her spirit. This year, I will be asking her friends who come to spend the evening of the 16th with me, to bring an unwrapped toy for a child, and I will be giving those to a charity to give to children in need for the holidays in her name.

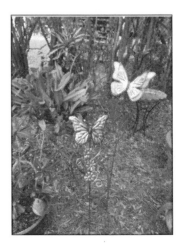

Additionally, across the yard, I planted a butterfly garden, so that there are always butterflies around her tree. In school I created a meditation garden for children to come and sit and read.

Some losses are especially painful and may turn your clients' world upside down, but you are there to guide and remind them of the resources they have and can use to heal and renew themselves. Observe how they view their world. It is positive or negative? How does this view impact the way they think of themselves?

Some of your clients may tell you they feel stuck—and they may not know they may be the ones holding themselves back.

❖

EXERCISE

• HEALING AND RENEWAL •

In what ways do you feel stuck?

_____

_____

What do you want to achieve as you rebuild your world?

_____

_____

Do you have control over your life?

_____

_____

What is holding you back?

_____

_____

What is preventing you from being happier?

_____

_____

Do you still allow your thoughts to have power over the quality of your life?

_____

_____

Many years ago I watched the movie *Circle of Iron*. It was metaphorical and involved martial arts in a mystical way. It was about overcoming obstacles, letting go of fears, and knowing oneself. In the movie, the warrior is looking for a wizard who has a book that contains all the answers of the world. When he meets the wizard, the warrior is given "the book of all knowledge." As he opens the book, all excited to find the answers, he gets a surprise. What he sees inside of the book is a mirror. In other words, the answers resided within himself.

You could show this movie to a group, followed by a discussion. Give them the following questions as a handout, and guide them to the answers within themselves and to finding meaning in their lives and rebuilding their world again.

Individual or Group Activities

EXERCISE

• FIND MEANING IN YOUR LIFE •

After watching *Circle of Iron*, how can you rebuild your world?

_____

_____

What answers have I been looking for outside myself?

_____

_____

As I connect with my inner self, I know that

_____

_____

> *The chances of finding the significance [for our surroundings] are always found in life; not even suffering and death can part us from that. ... Such recognition can renew the spiritual conscience of the individual in relation to their own divinity and value as a person.*
>
> — Melvin A. Kimble

Ask your clients about their purpose in **Life** and how each of the following applies to them:

- Transcendence
- Leaving a legacy: How do you want to be remembered?
- Embracing more love in my life: To give more love and open my heart to receive more love from others.
- Contributing to the world:
  Can you imagine touching the soul of someone?
- Compassion: For others and for myself

EXERCISE

• FINDING MEANING •

Grievers who choose transcendence recognize that they are not alone, that they share a common human condition, and that they are amongst so many who have experienced love and loss. They use their pain in a way that touches others. The pain is still there, of course, but it is transformed.

— Ashley Davis Bush

One way to look at this world is as a school for the soul. Your lifetime consists of experiences, tests, and lessons.

— Sharon Janis

As far as we can discern, the sole purpose of human existence is to kindle a light of meaning in the darkness of mere being.

— Carl Jung

How can you apply these quotes to find meaning?

Consider the life transition you have lived in recent times. Is there a life lesson in this experience?

Have you ever lived another major life transition?

How did you learn about yourself?

Can you mention a benefit that came out of that transition you didn't expect to happen?

Did your experience a have a positive outcome?

Did you grow as a person?

How can you apply this lesson of growth to the present situation?

What does this mean to you?

The affirmations are to be said with a sense of confidence, hope, and assurance every time your clients need a boost in the new phase of their transformation.

• AFFIRMATIONS •

Now, close your eyes and in your mind, repeat after me the following affirmations. Say these affirmations knowing you are able to rebuild your world with meaning. Make them your reality and be sure you can live a meaningful life.

- *I am able to rebuild my world.*
- *I am grateful for everything I have in my life.*
- *My life has meaning.*

Meditation

In this meditation your clients move closer and closer to their new world after picking up the pieces of their lives with all their love. They are able to find that determination and empowerment, inspired by meaning and gratitude.

• MEDITATION •

Find a comfortable position and very slowly close your eyes. Take a deep breath in and let it go. Take another deep breath and let it go. One more time, take a deep breath and let it go. Now, in your mind, repeat after me:

My world is fulfilled and has many possibilities. Within myself there is a rebirth and I have the capacity to rebuild my world with a higher meaning. I find meaning in every action I take and in each moment I live. Within myself there has been an inside-out transformation. My world is filled with blessings.

THERAPIST EXERCISE
• ARE YOU MEETING YOUR NEEDS? •

You have been doing a beautiful job guiding your clients into their personal transformation. You have given them the space to grieve, grow, and have hope for a brighter future. Now, it's your turn. Have you encountered a loss that shattered your world? Have you picked up the pieces or built a new foundation? If you did build the foundation, was it a foundation of a house made of straw or with bricks? This is your opportunity to start rebuilding your own world.

Do you know who you became after facing a major life transition?

_____

_____

Are you satisfied with the person you became, or are there areas in your life that need to be rebuilt?

_____

_____

How are you planning to do this rebuilding? Which strengths will you use?

_____

_____

Are you living according to your values?

_____

_____

Are you living your purpose?

_____

_____

The most important question: do you feel passionate for what you do?
Does it give meaning to your life?

_____

_____

Chapter 14

Principle XI: Visualize the Life You Want

> *Today brings you the opportunity to become a better person.*
> *Continue growing, and transform your life.*
>
> — Ligia M. Houben

When reaching this principle, your clients have completed *this* journey of transformation (as it continues evolving, it is a journey in process). The process started with accepting the loss and evolved into taking actions to embrace life again after that loss. In this principle you will explore different activities that will help your clients get closer to a happier and more meaningful life. As you go through this principle with your clients, you want to feel you have helped them transform their loss and, therefore, transform their lives.

Ask your clients how they see their lives in the future. They may have mixed emotions about keeping grief in their lives or embracing life again. They may feel ambivalent and unable to see that beautiful life in their future. You can help them, with these tools, get closer to that goal. We all want to be happy. Your clients want to be happy, even if they do not embrace that possibility yet. It is not about your feelings, it is about theirs. You only provide your help, your ideas, and your support. They make the choice. This is a good time to remind them of the drawing they did in Principle II, about the emotion they wanted to experience more often. They can move from taking baby steps to taking bigger steps as they walk their path.

Now, tell me, how do you see this emotion? • *How can you visualize your life feeling this way?*

DEFINITIONS OF VISUALIZING THE LIFE THEY WANT

I wish I could see a brighter future, but without my daughter it seems impossible. Will I change doing this? I want to live a life where I am helping mothers who lost children in a car accident. That is the life I want, I just don't know how to make it possible. What did you say I do? So, if I can imagine something in my mind, that is visualization?

I want to be happier. If this helps me, I will do it. Teach me how, as I do not have an idea how to do this.

— Definitions shared in seminars or by clients

Meaningful Quotes

> *What is the biggest lie in the world? It is: at a given moment*
> *of our existence we lose control of our lives, and it becomes governed by fate.*
> *This is the biggest lie in the world.*
>
> — Paulo Coelho, *The Alchemist*
>
> *The first step to carrying out a dream or change in you is desire.*
>
> — Napoleon Hill
>
> *Happiness depends upon ourselves.*
>
> — Aristotle
>
> *It doesn't matter how long we may have been stuck in a sense of our limitations. If we go*
> *into a darkened room and turn on the light, it doesn't matter if the room has been dark*
> *for a day, a week, or ten thousand years—we turn on the light and it is illuminated.*
> *Once we control our capacity for love and happiness, the light has been turned on.*
>
> — Unknown

❖

EXERCISE

• MEANINGFUL QUOTES •

What is a meaningful quote for you? Please write it below and then answer the following questions:

_____

What does this quote mean to you?

_____

How can you apply it?

_____

What is important about this quote?

_____

Would you have changed or deleted something from the quote? What? Why?

_____

Knowing Yourself

In order to visualize the world they want, your clients must know what they want. In order to know what they want, they must know themselves.

> ### *KNOW THYSELF*
>
> *Watch your thought; they become your words.*
> *Watch your words; they become your actions*
> *Watch your actions; they become your habits.*
> *Watch your habits; they become your character.*
> *Watch your character for it will become your destiny.*
>
> — Hillel

After reading Hillel's words, ask your clients to write (for the second time), "WHO AM I?" The difference is that after going through the process of transformation, they can see who they are now and how they want to be in the future.

Self-Evalution

If clients are confused and need to explore who they really are at this point in their lives, ask them to answer the following questions:

- What words come to your mind when you think about yourself?
- What do you want?
- What type of activities are you doing on a regular basis?
- Who are your friends? Are they understanding or judgmental?
- Are you an active or sedentary person?
- Are you religious or spiritual? How do you connect with your inner self?
- What types of books, films, or music do you enjoy?
- Do you like to travel? Which country or city would you like to visit?
- How would you like to see yourself professionally? Do you want to change your career?
- What do you like to wear? What do you like to eat? How do you like to relax?

After they respond to these questions, ask them to compose an essay inspired by their answers.

EXERCISE
• WHO DO I WANT TO BE? •

After getting in touch with your essence and knowing who you are now, you may realize there are areas in your life you want to improve. Describe those areas:

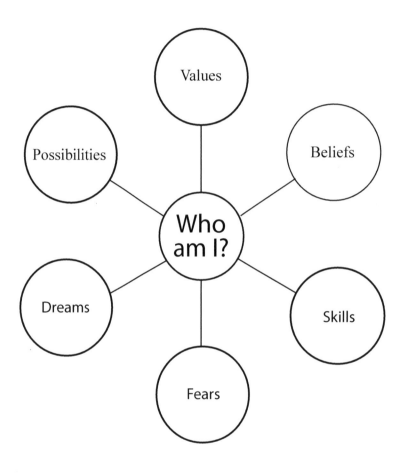

_____

_____

_____

_____

_____

_____

EXERCISE

• LIFE ASSESSMENT •

In order to have your ideal life and become the person you want to be, the first step you need to take is doing an honest assessment of your reality. Start by evaluating each of your life dimensions.

On a scale from 1 to 10, rate different areas of your life:

Physical (includes health and wellness)_____

Emotional (includes loving relationships)_____

Social (includes friends, colleagues, and people in general)_____

Spiritual (includes religion, if applicable, and connectedness)_____

List two things you CAN do to improve your physical dimension:

    1._____

    2._____

List two things you CAN do to improve your emotional dimension:

    1._____

    2._____

List two things you CAN do to improve your social dimension:

    1._____

    2._____

List two things you CAN do to improve your spiritual dimension:

    1._____

    2._____

List two things you CAN do to improve your financial dimension:

    1._____

    2._____

List two things you CAN do to improve your professional dimension:

    1._____

    2._____

List two things you CAN do to improve your personal growth dimension:

    1._____

    2._____

How would your life benefit once you take action in all these dimensions?

Is Happiness a Choice?

If your clients constantly think they cannot be happy again, you can share with them the words of the Dalai Lama, "Happiness is not something readymade. It comes from your own actions."

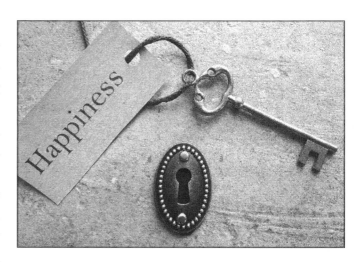

The happiness of your clients will depend on the actions they take. It has to come from within, and it takes time and effort. However, if they want to be happy, they need to take actions to make it a reality. Because happiness is subjective, start by asking your client how they define happiness and whether they think it is a choice.

Attitude and Happiness

Being happy is a choice and it has to do with attitude. Your clients can choose to be happier based on their attitude and the things they are doing.

How is Your Attitude in Life?

Their attitude greatly influences how your clients see life after a loss and whether they want to take actions to feel happier. You may want to share with them what Bernie Siegel (2005) says, "Maintaining a positive attitude, no matter what your circumstances, increases the likelihood of your finding future happiness and fulfillment".

> **Individual or Group Activities**
>
>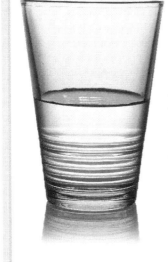
>
> **STRATEGY**
>
> ### • Glass Half Full or Half Empty •
>
> Show your clients this picture and ask them how they see the glass.
>
> Allow them to elaborate on their response and how this response affects their attitude.
>
> For a group setting, place a full water pitcher on a table with several empty glasses. Then, ask the members of the group to pour themselves a glass of water based on how they see life. If they happen to leave the glass empty or half empty, ask them to mention positive things they can start doing that reflects taking care of themselves. For each positive action, little by little, they could fill up the glass. It is about empowering them to have a healthier, happier life.

STRATEGY

• DISCOVER YOUR ATTITUDE IN LIFE •

How do you see life? If you change your attitude you can change your life.

1. Each day brings a new opportunity.

2. I can better the quality of my life.

3. Life is beautiful.

4. Life is only problems.

5. Most people are good.

6. Most people have bad intentions.

7. I cannot say no.

8. I always say no.

9. I don't take time to examine my life.

10. I ignore what I feel.

11. I don't know where I am going.

12. My life is balanced.

13. My life needs a review.

14. I don't care about others.

15. Life is so difficult.

16. Everything goes wrong.

17. Life is a gift.

18. I can change my life.

19. I leave things to chance.

20. I am ready to transform my life.

EXERCISE

• DO YOU WANT TO BE HAPPY? •

Are you struggling with the desire to be happier but do not know how? Allow hope to enter your life and to guide in building a brighter future. Give yourself permission to be happy again, to hope, and to live a life with meaning. It can be done. You can do it! If you think it is possible to transform your loss, you will! It all starts with believing in you.

Define happiness:

_____

_____

Do you think you can create your own happiness?

_____

_____

Become a happier version of yourself.

Finish the following sentences:

Life is:

_____

_____

My life is:

_____

_____

The most important thing in my life is:

_____

_____

Bring More Happiness into Your Life

Sharon Janis (2000) has one of the simplest "recipes" to be happy. She states that the following efforts can help you become a happier person:

Hope for the best.
Shoot for the best.
Expect the best.
Be perfectly content with whatever comes.

Ask your client to do the following exercise to evaluate how often they are doing things they enjoy. During the exercise play relaxing music, light a candle, and invite clients to reflect on their responses. The purpose is to focus on happiness.

In addition to listing things that make them happy, clients could make a picture collage of things that could bring them happiness.

❖
EXERCISE

• THESE THINGS MAKE ME HAPPY •

Write a list of the things that make you happy and review how many of them you actually do.

These things make me happy	How often I do this	How often I want to do it
1.		
2.		
3.		
4.		
5.		

KEY _____

W: Weekly • **D:** Daily • **M:** Monthly • **S:** Seldom • **N:** Never

STRATEGY

• COMMITMENT WITH THEMSELVES •

Not surprisingly, your clients often are not doing ANYTHING that brings them happiness. If this is the case, ask them to write a contract with themselves:

I commit that every single day I will do something that brings joy to my life.

Signature   Date

_____   _____

HAPPINESS AND GRATITUDE

Happiness lies deep within us, in the very core of our being.
Happiness does not exist in any external object, but only in us,
who are the consciousness that experiences happiness.
Though we seem to derive happiness from external objects or experiences,
the happiness that we thus enjoy in fact arises from within us.

— Sri Ramana

Is there a connection between happiness and being grateful? Is it when you are happy that you are grateful, or vice versa? In Principle III, we expanded in the concept of gratitude. Now, we link it to happiness.

The following suggestions can be shared with your clients in the form of a handout.

Strategy

• Be Happy •

In Order To Be Happy, Stop Doing This:
- Focusing on your shortcomings or challenges
- Dwelling on your pain
- Comparing yourself with others
- Complaining about your misfortune
- Keeping anger, jealousy, or envy in your heart
- Saying how unhappy you are
- Blaming, complaining, and procrastinating

Instead, Do This:
- Be grateful for what you have
- Know your gifts/talents
- Follow your dream
- Focus on your goals and take action
- Visualize the life you want on a regular basis

• Visualization on Happiness •

Close your eyes and imagine a beautiful place. Call this place happyworld. In this place you feel a sense a complete joy. How is this place? Imagine it vividly. As you see it in your mind and see yourself happy, believe you CAN be happy. Pay attention to your surroundings. What colors do you see? What do you smell? What do you hear?

Now, make the colors brighter, the smells stronger, and the sounds louder, but still pleasant to the ear. You feel a great joy inside. You feel complete. You feel fulfilled. You are happy. Feel that emotion and make it stronger. Allow this sensation of happiness to radiate from your heart and expand to every cell in your body. Embrace this emotion deeply in your being, take a deep breath in, and as you exhale, open your eyes.

LIVING YOUR MEANINGFUL LIFE

What the mind can conceive and believe, the mind can achieve.

— Napoleon Hill

After your clients have evaluated where they are in life, the areas they want to improve, and the desire to be happier, they can start the creation process. Moving forward after a loss means they have discovered there is life after a loss and they have accepted their new reality.

The can create a purposeful and meaningful life after their loss.

Ask them to answer the following questions:

- *Are you living the life you want?*
- *Are you following your dream?*
- *Do you have a purpose in life?*

As you work with this principle you can help clients to write a mission statement that involves intention, focus, and purpose for a meaningful life.

• CREATING YOUR MEANINGFUL LIFE •

As you engage in this exercise, I want you to feel relaxed. Start by taking a deep breath in and after letting it out, think the following phrase: *I want to live a life with meaning. I am able to live a life with meaning. I can create a life with meaning.* Take another deep breath and open your eyes.

Now, begin writing your mission statement about the life you want. A mission statement is a phrase that includes your values, purpose in life, and reason for existing in this world.

Life is:

_____

_____

My life is:

_____

_____

The most important thing in my life is:

_____

_____

My purpose in life is:

_____

_____

My main values are:

_____

_____

My mission statement is:

_____

_____

Goal Setting with Purpose

As your clients begin setting goals, you want them to focus on their strengths. You want them to remember they have inner resources to live the life they desire.

❖

EXERCISE

• STRENGTHS AND GOALS •

Is there a specific strength you need in order to make a reality your ideal life?

At this point, go back to Principle I and enumerate your strengths. After this, choose one of *these* strengths that would help you the most at this moment in time.

What strengths do you have?

1. _____

2. _____

3. _____

4. _____

5. _____

6. _____

When have you felt strong or used any of these strengths? _____

_____

Go to that moment now and recreate those feelings. Make the colors bright, maybe you can add some energized music to it!

Remember what words have helped you. If you feel stuck in your process it may be that a limiting thought is in your mind. Stop now and list thoughts you may have on a regular basis that are delaying your growing process. Then answer the following questions:

What excuses will I let go of? _____

What thoughts will I modify? _____

• WRITE A LETTER OF STRENGTH •

Write a letter to yourself listing all the strength you have, how you have used them in the past, and how these strength will help you now in your transformation. Give it to a person you trust who loves you and ask that person to mail it to you in three months.

Ten things you want to have, be, or do:

1. _____

2. _____

3. _____

4. _____

5. _____

6. _____

7. _____

8. _____

9. _____

10. _____

If you find yourself holding on to limiting beliefs, this is the time to let them go. Replace them with the thoughts, "I deserve happiness. I am able to be happy."

In order to go somewhere, to any destination, it is necessary to have a direction. If do not know how to get there, you may use a map, GPS, or phone call.

You need to know where you are going and how to get there. The same happens in life.

Transformation is not something you attain. It is an outcome based on actions. It is an intersection where the body, mind, and spirit all come together.

The most wonderful part is that at any time, you can start making different choices and different decisions, taking different steps and inevitably arriving at a different place from where you are today.

Think about three roadblocks you have encountered on this journey and that have kept you from moving forward. You may need to let them go for growth to happen.

Your clients may have tried to achieve goals in the past and not succeeded. They may have gotten into a pattern that sabotages their purpose. They may focus on their obstacles rather than their goals. Now is the time to break the cycle. Ask them to review the following diagram and see if they have found themselves in this loop in the past. Have them answer the questions that follow.

❖

EXERCISE

• FINDING YOUR PURPOSE •

Fear, Anger
Anxiety, Depression,
Insecurity

Evaluation, Realization,
Decision, Possibilities

Fear About
The future

Goals, Plan Of Action,
Execution, New Life

Do you have any of these challenges that keep you from achieving your goals?

- Lack of clarity
- Lack of organization
- Lack of trust

- Lack of focus
- Procrastination

How can you overcome each of the challenges you selected?_____

Describe how you want to be living your life in the future: How do you see your life in a year or two? How would you have contributed to humanity, with your family or your own life? Have you left a legacy? What goals would you have achieved?

GOAL _____

GOAL _____

GOAL _____

EXERCISE

• QUALITIES OF AN IDEAL PERSON •

Which of the following qualities would help you take action to achieve the life you want? Then, think about a person (living, dead, or imaginary) who has such qualities and keep this image in your mind.

Courage	Love	Resilience
Faith	Hope	Optimism
Patience	Discipline	Strength
Determination	Honesty	Perseverance

Other:

_____

_____

_____

Imagine you are sitting in a movie theater. The curtains are closed. Then, you see in the movie the person with the qualities chosen from the above list doing what you wish you could do. Then, the screen goes blank and the curtains close. Now, the curtains open again and the film playing is you doing the things you wish to do, embracing the qualities of the other person. Now, the screen goes blank. The curtains close. Finally, the curtains open again and you ARE in the film, doing what you saw yourself doing, feeling empowered and making it a reality.

STRATEGY

• THE TWO CHAIRS •

For this activity you need two chairs, one next to the other. Ask your client to sit on the first chair and ask them to close their eyes. Now, say these words:

Imagine yourself a year from now feeling the same way you are feeling now. (In the case of your client, you know his or her story, so you include what has been happening.)

You have remained angry, unable to forgive, and sad. You find yourself in a dark place. You have not been able to feel better and you are sad all the time. You are always complaining. You have not been able to rebuild your world and you feel stuck. Make those emotions stronger and stronger. Now, open your eyes and shake your body.

Then, ask your client to move to the second chair. Now say these words:

Imagine yourself in a year from now feeling happier, being able to live with meaning, and feeling grateful for what you have in your life. See yourself peaceful, relaxed, and joyful. Feel how great you feel after having contributed to humanity with your actions, with your love, with your care. Now, make those emotions stronger. See it vividly. See the colors brighter and brighter and hold in your heart how happy you feel! Now, open your eyes.

Tell me, which chair do you prefer?

Because the power of this exercise is that they will be able to experience the different emotions, 10 out of 10 times, they will tell you they prefer the second chair. The beauty is that it is their choice.

After setting goals, focusing on strengths, and feeling empowered, your clients will have the opportunity to visualize their lives in a graphic manner. They will be able to create their ideal! You can ask clients to do this exercise at home and bring you the vision board, or to do it as an engaging and motivating group activity.

EXERCISE

• CREATING A VISION BOARD •
OF YOUR IDEAL LIFE

The following materials are needed for this exercise:

Cardboard or poster board   Photos
Scissors   Scanned images
Glue   Stickers
Magazines   Marker
Newspapers

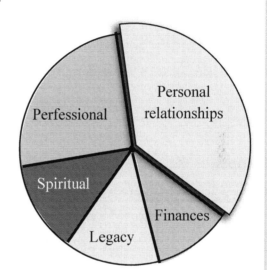

This vision board will enable you to visualize your goals with purpose and meaning. Begin by placing a photo of yourself in the center of the board. Remember to include the most important areas of your life.

- Physical   • Emotional
- Spiritual   • Social
- Relationships   • Financial

Now, cut pictures from magazines, newspapers, photos, or scan images from the computer. You may also integrate words or phrases that will help you stay focused and motivated. Do not be afraid to be creative. Use your imagination. Visualize and manifest your ideal life.

Enjoy it! The purpose of this meaningful project is to stimulate your imagination and creativity so you can visualize the life you want.

Place the vision board somewhere you will see it often. Whenever you find yourself lacking hope or motivation, you can look at it and remind yourself of the ideal life you are striving for.

You are able to create your life. You can do it!
Remember, our lives have meaning and, as you transform your loss, you transform your life!

• AFFIRMATIONS •

These affirmations are said in an empowered, hopeful, and self-confident manner. They can say them out loud in front of a mirror every morning.

Now, close your eyes and in your mind, repeat after me the following affirmations. Say these affirmations in an empowered way and make them your reality. You may write them down on a blank card and carry them with you.

- *My life is meaningful and I am in charge of it.*
- *I can build the life I desire.*
- *I am ready to achieve my goals.*
- *I deserve to be happy.*

Meditation

This is the final meditation. At this point, hopefully your clients have embraced this practice and have discovered the benefits it brings to their lives. Remind them to continue practicing on a regular basis as they continue living centered, relaxed, and with joy in their hearts.

• MEDITATION•

Find a comfortable position and very slowly close your eyes. Take a deep breath in and let it go. Take another deep breath and let it go. One more time, take a deep breath and let it go. Now, in your mind, repeat after me:

My life is a gift and it has great meaning. I understand that my happiness is the result of my decisions and how I relate to myself and others. Therefore, I choose to be happy. By transforming my loss, I have acquired the ability to build a life with a greater purpose. I thank God for my life and for giving me the ability to love and feel.

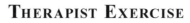

THERAPIST EXERCISE

• ARE YOU HAPPY? •

In this final principle, you have explored different ways your clients can build a brighter future. They went through the process of transformation and are ready to visualize the life they want. It is the last principle and the beginning of their new lives. There is life after loss, and you have helped your client embrace it. Thank you! Now, what about your life? I hope this last principle (as the previous ones) has helped you to realize that happiness is a choice and you also want to be HAPPY! If you are already doing things to be happy, great! If not, start NOW to make it a reality. Life is a gift and just as you taught your clients, unwrap it with love and care.

How do you define happiness?

_____

_____

Are you happy?

_____

How are your life dimensions?

On a scale from 1 to 10, rate each of your life dimensions:

Physical _____

Emotional _____

Social _____

Spiritual _____

What activities do you engage in that bring joy to your life?

_____

_____

How can living with joy and purpose help when working with clients?

_____

_____

Chapter 15

What About You?

We have come to the end of our journey. We have explored together different ways to help your clients transform their loss and transform their lives. Now, what about you?

As I said at the beginning, it all starts with you. Continue being that special human being you are as you accompany and guide your clients in their process. Continue to pay attention to your own needs and to transforming your own life. Remember to:

- Be centered and connected with your inner self.
- Allow yourself some "me-time."
- Engage in some physical activity.
- Meditate with breathing techniques.
- Do some journaling.
- Share time with others.
- And, in case you haven't done it, transform your OWN loss!

I leave you with the inspiring words of Mahatma Gandhi:

Be the change you want to see in the world.

FINAL REFLECTION

Writing this book has been a journey. A beautiful journey, I must say! I had the concept in my mind for some years, but because of a personal loss I experienced January of 2014, when I was hit by a car while crossing the street, I had to put my project on hold. To my delightful surprise, Linda Jackson proposed I write a workbook for PESI based on my seminar, *Transforming Grief and Loss: Strategies to Help Your Clients Through Major Loss*. What a joy this was!

I have written this book with my heart.

I hope you embrace it with an open mind and open heart, and use it as a meaningful tool in your practice, as you continue your own journey.

Thank you for being you!

REFERENCES

❖

```
For your convenience, you may download a PDF version of the exercises in this book
from our dedicated website: go.pesi.com/grief
```

Adams, C. (2003). ABC's of Grief: A Handbook for Survivors. Amityville, NY: Baywood Publishing Company.

Adler, Alfred. (2014). What Life Could Mean to You (Timeless Wisdom Collection Book 196) Kindle Edition. Business and Leadership Publishing.

Amen, Daniel G. (1999). Change Your Brain, Change Your Life. New York, NY: Three Rivers Press.

Andreas, S. & Faulkner, C. (1995). NLP: The New Technology of Achievement. New York: Morrow.

Attig, Thomas. (2010). How We Grieve: Relearning the World, 2nd ed. Oxford University Press.

Becker, E. (2001). Loss and Growth: The Grief Spiral: Transformative Bereavement. Key West, FL: Whiz Bang LLC.

Borysenko, Joan. (1990). Guilt Is the Teacher, Love Is the Lesson. New York: Warner Books, 175.

Bradbury, A. (2006). Develop Your NLP Skills, 3rd ed. London: Kogan Page.

Browne, S. (2006). Light a Candle. Cincinnati, OH: Angel Bea Publishing.

Byock, Ira. (2014). The Four Things That Matter Most: A Book About Living. Atria Books.

Campbell, Joseph. (2008). The Collected Works of Joseph Campbell, 3rd ed. New World Library.

Complete Guide to Pilates, Yoga, Meditation & Stress Relief. (2002). Bath: Paragon.

Christian Conte. (2009). Advanced Technologies for Counseling and Psychotherapy. New York: Springer Publishing Company, LLC.

Chopra, Deepak. (1994). The Seven Spiritual Laws of Success: A Practical Guide to the Fulfillment of Your Dreams. New World Library/Amber-Allen Publishing.

Coelho, Paulo. (1993). The Alchemist. HarperCollins.

Conte, Christian. (2009). Advanced Techniques for Counseling and Psychotherapy. Springer Publishing Company.

Corey, M. & Corey, G. (1992). Groups: Process and Practice, 4th ed. Pacific Grove, CA: Brooks/Cole Pub.

Coriat, H. Isador. (2015). The Meaning of Dreams. Forgotten Books.

Doige, Norman. (2007). The Brain That Changes Itself: Stories of Personal Triumph from the Frontiers of Brain Science. Penguin Books.

Doka, J. Kenneth & Martin, L. Terry. (1999). Men Don't Cry, Women Do: Transcending Gender Stereotypes of Grief. Routledge.

Doka, J. Kenneth & Martin, L. Terry. (2010). Grieving Beyond Gender: Understanding the Ways Men and Women Mourn, rev. ed. New York: Routledge.

Epstein, G. (1989). Healing Visualizations: Creating Health Through Imagery. New York: Bantam Books.

Hay, L. & Kessler, D. (2014). You Can Heal Your Heart: Finding Peace After a Breakup, Divorce, or Death, 2nd ed. Hay House.

Helmstetter, Shad. (1987). What to Say When You Talk to Yourself. New York: Simon & Schuster.

Helmstetter, Shad. (2014). The Power of Neuroplasticity. CreateSpace Independent Publishing Platform.

Hewapathirane, Daya. (2013). Mindfulness Movement in the Western World. http://www.lankaweb. com/news/items/2013/06/06/mindfulness-movement-in-the-western-world/.

Hope, J. (2001). The Meditation Year. North Adams, MA: Storey Books.

Houben, Ligia M. (2006). Spirituality and Aging: The Fourth Dimension.

Imber-Black, Evan & Roberts, Janine. (1998). Rituals for Our Times: Celebrating, Healing, and Changing Our Lives and Our Relationships (Master Work Series). Jason Aronson, Inc.

James, Allen. (2014). As a Man Thinketh. CreateSpace Independent Publishing Platform.

James, Allen (2014). James Allen's Book of Meditations for Every Day in the Year. CreateSpace Independent Publishing Platform.

Janis, Sharon. (2008). Spirituality for Dummies, 2nd ed. For Dummies.

Kabat-Zinn, Jon. (2006). Mindfulness for Beginners. Sounds True, Inc.

Kauffman, Jeffrey. (2002). Loss of the Assumptive World: A Theory of Traumatic Loss. Routledge.

Kornfield, Jack. (2008). Meditation for Beginners. Sounds True, Inc.

Lesowitz, N. & Sammons, M. (2009). Living Life As a Thank You: The Transformative Power of Gratitude. San Francisco: Viva Editions.

Noble, Marty. (2013). Creative Haven Tibetan Designs Coloring Book. Dover Publications.

Rasheed, Janice M., Rasheed, Mikal N. & Marley James A. (2010). Family Therapy: Models and Techniques. Thousand Oaks, CA: Sage.

Samuels, M. (1990). Healing with the Mind's Eye: How to Use Guided Imagery and Visions to Heal Body, Mind, and Spirit, rev. ed. Hoboken, NJ: John Wiley & Sons.

Sarno, John E. (2007). The Divided Mind: The Epidemic of Mindbody Disorders. HarperCollins.

Schwartz, Jeffrey M. (2003). The Mind and the Brain: Neuroplasticity and the Power of Mental Force. Harper Perennial

Siegel, B. (2005). 101 Exercises for the Soul: A Divine Workout Plan for Body, Mind, and Spirit. Novato, CA: New World Library.

Southwick, M. Steven & Charney, S. Dennis. (2012). Resilience: The Science of Mastering Life's Greatest Challenges. Cambridge University Press.

Wilson, J. (2014). Supporting People Through Loss and Grief: An Introduction for Counsellors and Other Caring Practitioners. Jessica Kingsley Publishers.

Winokuer, H., & Harris, D. (2012). Principles and Practice of Grief Counseling. New York: Springer.

Wolfelt, Alan D. (2004). The Understanding Your Grief Journal: Exploring the Ten Essential Touchstones. Companion Press.

Worden, J. (1982). Grief Counseling and Grief Therapy: A Handbook for the Mental Health Practitioner, 4th ed. New York: Springer.

WEBSITE REFERENCES

❖

Pauline Boss
www.ambiguousloss.com

Center for Complicated Grief
www.complicatedgrief.org/bereavement

David Kessler
www.grief.com

Role Play
www.engadet.com

Therapy In Color
www.therapyincolor.tumblr.com

Prayers
www.prayers-for-special-help.com

Neuro-Linguistic Programming (NLP)
www.lightworkseminar.com

Song Lyrics
www.metrolyrics.com

Grief Blogs
www.griefhealingblog.com
www.hellogrief.org
www.griefrecoverymethod.com/blog
www.grieflink.com
www.ligiahouben.blogspot.com

Food Planner
www.foodplannerapp.com

Ostrich Pillow
www.studiobananthings.com

The 11 Principles of Transformation
http://ligiahouben.com/the-11-principles-of-transformation/

Made in the USA
Columbia, SC
05 November 2021

48394529R00146